The Alchemy of Fasting

Explore Intermittent Fasting for Health and Self-Discovery

Luca Danton

Copyright © 2024 by Luca Danton

All rights reserved. No part of this publication may be reproduced, distributed, or transmitted in any form or by any means, including photocopying, recording, or other electronic or mechanical methods, without the prior written permission of the author, except in the case of brief quotations embodied in critical reviews and certain other noncommercial uses permitted by copyright law.

The Alchemy of Fasting:

Explore Intermittent Fasting for Health and Self-Discovery

Luca Danton

Independently Published

2024

ISBN: 978-99922-2-855-5

☼

"Alchemy is the process of changing lead into gold. Inner alchemy (personal transformation) occurs when we clear our clutter—internal and external—and let go of things that no longer serve us well. This creates balance and space, a place that fosters contentment and joy."
- Laurie Buchanan

Contents

1 The Quest Begins With US — 7

2 Fasting Myths And You — 17

3 Listening To Our Bodies — 33

4 Emotional Hunger Vs. Physical Hunger — 47

5 Fueling Your Fasted Workouts — 62

6 Stress, Anxiety, And Our Inner Calm — 72

7 Fasting, Sleep, And Food Choices — 94

8 Finding Your Middle Way — 109

1
The Quest Begins With US

Food. It has been my greatest love and my most challenging adversary. From the moment I first discovered the joys of taste and texture, I was hooked. The sizzle of a perfectly seared steak, the velvety smoothness of a rich chocolate mousse, the crisp snap of a fresh apple - these were the simple pleasures that made life worth living. But this love affair has also been a complicated one, fraught with cycles of overindulgence, digestive discomfort and the nagging sense that my relationship with nourishment was out of balance.

Let me be clear: the mere thought of eating food I do not want or like is not appealing to me. This doesn't mean that I only eat junk food or sweets, far from it. I enjoy a salad as well as the next guy, but please, do not give me salads all week long! I believe life is a balance, and this should be reflected in your meals also. Food intake is closely related to my mood. Give me food that is not appealing to me or restrict the quantities to where I'm still hungry and my mood suffers. I can easily become insufferable, hunger and anxiety do me in.

I like food, I simply do, I like eating, preparing, cooking, and also shopping for it. I have no issue with preparing food or doing the dishes afterward. My mother had me help her around the kitchen when I was a kid and my wife is a chef, although she doesn't work in the food industry any more, so it is better for me since I'm on the receiving end of her creations. Food is one of the passions of my life.

This passion for food led me to overeat. Something about the taste of fresh pasta with a little tomatoes cut in cubes with minced basil that kept me coming back for "Just a little more, this is it I promise! I was popping Tums like they were M&Ms at times. All this enjoyment of food had its consequences, especially after 40. I have had the pleasure of being acquainted with the Prazole family: Lansoprazole, Omeprazole, Esomeprazole, Rabeprazole, I know them well enough to be on a first name basis with them. I took them daily without respite, or suffer the consequences.

For years, I found myself caught in an endless loop of overeating the foods I craved, only to be met with unpleasant consequences – bloating, acid reflux, and a general heaviness that seemed to weigh me down both physically and mentally. I would try to break free through restrictive diets, only to find myself rebounding back to my old habits, the deprivation often leading to a sense of unease and resentment. All this suffering and distress to reach a much-desired target weight that the scale sometimes conceded, and sometimes not. Usually the deprivation of my favorite foods led me back to them with a vengeance, it was a matter of time until the scale went back to where it usually sits.

Can you relate to this? Have you ever found yourself trapped in the endless loop of yo-yo dieting, desperate for a way out but unsure of where to turn? I know I have. For years, I convinced myself that if I just had more willpower, more discipline, I could break free from this pattern of self-harm. But the truth is, it was never about the food itself. It was about the way I was using food to numb my emotions, to distract myself from the deeper issues that lurked beneath the surface.

Something had to change. I knew I was overweight because I overate, but I dreaded the idea of going on a diet because it made me quite irritable and anxious. I have exercised regularly throughout my life, I do about 30 minutes to an hour of exercise daily. I'm no athlete, but I move my body regularly. I could try to extend my daily workout, but could I keep this up for a long period of time? I'm 53 now, after the age of 45 I began to notice that exercise is necessary for your body. For me, it is more about keeping your body's strength and flexibility for your later years than trying to break a record. I respect immensely everyone that runs a marathon after 50, but I'm not sure if it's a road I want to go down on.

Despite my regular exercise routine, I found myself stuck in a vicious cycle. I knew my overeating habits were the root cause of my weight gain, but the thought of restrictive diets filled me with dread. I had experienced the irritability and anxiety that came with depriving myself of the foods I enjoyed, and I feared that any attempt to change my eating habits would only lead to more frustration and disappointment.

I was caught in an endless loop of overeating the foods I like, feeling bloated, acid reflux, feeling my body a bit heavy and slow because it was processing all the food I overate. Only after discovering fasting did I realize that I had been eating dinner for decades without being hungry. It's just something I did. When the kids where young we sat down to the table for dinner and breakfast, because it was family time and everybody had a chance to catch up and talk about their day. Nobody can argue about the benefits of sharing a meal with family, especially when you are raising your young children. I ate out of routine, not hunger. It was almost mechanical. The next day, I would eat breakfast, not hungry at all.

It was a familiar pattern, one that I'm sure you can relate to. The scale would fluctuate, my clothes would fit tighter and looser, and I would oscillate between moments of triumph and utter frustration. I knew that something had to change, but the idea of going on yet another diet filled me with dread. The mere thought of having to subsist on foods that didn't truly satisfy me was enough to make me want to throw in the towel before I even began.

You see, it wasn't just about the weight for me. It was about finding a way to break free from the cycle of overeating, digestive discomfort, and the nagging feeling that my body and mind were out of sync. I had always prided myself on being relatively active, with a daily exercise routine that kept my body moving. But even that didn't seem to be enough to counteract the effects of my haphazard eating habits.

A Sunday afternoon I was scrolling through Youtube videos when I stumbled upon on a Dr. Fung video on intermittent fasting. It was a talk uploaded on March 10th, 2016 about the two compartment problem. The video piqued my interest and led me to further investigate the issue. Watch it in your spare time if you are so inclined. I'm not a doctor or nutritionist, having said that, with my limited knowledge on science but with a vast knowledge on how my body feels and functions; I decided to further investigate and maybe give a try and see what happens.

As I explored intermittent fasting further, I was intrigued by the idea of giving my body a chance to rest and reset, to allow my digestive system to complete its natural cycles without the constant influx of new food. The notion of a 12-hour fasting window, from 8 pm to 8 am, didn't seem too daunting—after all, I was already asleep for a good portion of that time.

And so I embarked on this journey of self-discovery, armed with nothing but my own determination and a willingness to listen to my body's cues. In the beginning, it was a struggle. I would find myself watching the clock, counting down the minutes until I could break my fast. But slowly, something began to shift. I started to notice the difference between true hunger and emotional cravings. I began to appreciate the way my body felt when it was given the chance to fully process and assimilate the nutrients I was consuming.

The 8pm cutoff time led to a discovery I wasn't privy of before, why did I have the need to snack after dinner? Was I really hungry? No, I was not. I ate to appease my mind. But why? Why did I desire gratification? What need of mine was I fulfilling with these snacking? I mean, the human body can go for days without food, I was sure my life was not in danger for fasting 12 hours, but somehow I felt uneasy by having to not eat for a specific amount of time.

You see, I wasn't actually hungry. The urge to keep eating, to seek that gratification, wasn't driven by a physical need for nourishment. It was something deeper, a psychological and emotional craving that I had been feeding for years without even realizing it. As I sat with the discomfort of not being able to indulge this habitual behavior, I found myself questioning the nature of my hunger—was it truly physical, or was it something else entirely?

As I said, it is not that I was hungry, because I was not. I had this urge to eat something. I discovered tea. Somehow, the warmth of tea going down and warming my stomach made me cope better with the fasting time schedule.

Slowly, I started to extend my fasting window, pushing the boundaries of what I had once thought possible. With each passing day, I discovered more about the intricate workings of my body and the complex interplay between physical, emotional, and psychological factors when it came to my relationship with food.

I learned that I digest food quite slowly, and that adding more food to my body before the previous meal had been fully processed often left me feeling bloated, sluggish, and prone to acid reflux. I discovered that certain foods, like garlic, had a particularly pronounced effect on my digestion, causing me discomfort in a way that I had never fully appreciated before.

Perhaps most significantly, I began to notice a shift in my emotional and mental state as I adapted to this new way of nourishing myself. My "hanger" was subdued, since I identified those feelings in my body with anxiety instead of hunger. It made me look inward to find the source of my anxiety. I was more aware of my feelings, because I could correctly identify that the source of my discomfort was not hunger, but something else. I was no longer just reacting to physical cues but learning to listen to the deeper signals my body was sending me.

As I became more attuned to the nuances of my hunger,

I found that I was able to better discern when I was truly in need of nourishment and when I was seeking comfort or distraction through food. This newfound self-knowledge was empowering, allowing me to make more mindful choices about what and when I ate, rather than simply operating on autopilot.

In a way, this journey of intermittent fasting has been as much about self-discovery as it has been about dietary change. With each passing day, I've peeled back another layer of the complex relationship I've had with food, uncovering truths about my body, my emotions, and the ways in which the two are inextricably linked.

It's important to remember that fasting is not a one siz fits all prescription. What works for one person may not necessarily work for the next. Fasting is more of a journey in which one listens to the body, learns the difference between physical hunger and the constant need for immediate gratification, and finds a balanced approach that supports overall well-being. For some, a 12-hour fasting window may be the sweet spot, while others may thrive on longer fasting periods. The key is to approach this exploration with an open mind, patience, and a willingness to adapt as you gain a deeper understanding of your own unique needs and rhythms.

This journey isn't about adhering to a rigid, universal formula, but about embarking on a deeply personal exploration – one that requires us to listen closely to the wisdom of our bodies, to uncover the roots of our emotional connections to food, and to find the balance that allows us to nourish ourselves in a way that truly supports our overall health and happiness.

And now, as I invite you to join me on this transformative quest, I want you to know that you are not alone. I know that the challenges I've faced – the cycles of overeating, the frustration with dieting, the nagging sense that something is off – are not unique to me. They are the shared experiences of so many individuals who are seeking a more harmonious, sustainable path to well-being.

So, if any of this resonates with you, I encourage you to keep reading. Let's embark on this quest together, sharing our stories, our insights, and our discoveries along the way. For in the end, the true value of this exploration lies not in the act of fasting itself, but in the profound personal growth and self-awareness that can emerge when we approach our relationship with food with curiosity, compassion, and a willingness to challenge our preconceptions.

The journey begins here, with us. Let's dive in.

2
Fasting Myths And You

As I dove into the world of intermittent fasting, I quickly realized that there were numerous misconceptions and myths surrounding this transformative practice. These preconceptions had long deterred me from even considering fasting as a viable option for improving my health and well-being. In fact, the mere thought of depriving myself of food for extended periods filled me with a sense of dread and anxiety, a reaction born out of my past experiences with restrictive dieting.

You see, I had been down that road before, the endless cycle of yo-yo dieting that left me feeling deprived, frustrated, and ultimately, no closer to feeling comfortable and content with my food intake and weight. The memory of those restrictive regimes, where I would dutifully deny myself the foods I loved, only to inevitably cave and binge, was still fresh in my mind. The emotional turmoil, the irritability, the constant battle with my own willpower - it was a battle I had fought time and time again, only to emerge frustrated, my self-confidence shaken.

So, when I first stumbled upon the concept of intermittent fasting, I'll admit, I was skeptical. Wasn't this just another form of deprivation, another diet that would leave me feeling hungry and miserable? Surely, I couldn't possibly reap any benefits from intermittent fasting. These preconceptions had long deterred me from even considering fasting as a viable option for improving my health and well-being. In fact, the mere thought of depriving myself of food for extended periods filled me with a sense of dread and anxiety, a reaction born out of my past experiences with restrictive dieting.

Exploring the research and personal accounts of those who had embraced this lifestyle helped me see things in a new light. The more I learned, the more I realized that my preconceptions about fasting were not only misguided but also potentially hindering my path to true well-being.

I am not a doctor and this is not medical advice. I only share my experiences with fasting so you can have enough elements to make a decision about intermittent fasting yourself. Prior to starting intermittent fasting, I was in generally good health, aside from the persistent acid reflux and indigestion I experienced. I was generally healthy, with no major health issues. My yearly checkups showed no concerning problems, and I was in good overall physical condition prior to starting intermittent fasting.

It's time to shatter these myths and uncover the truth about fasting - a practice that, when approached with an open mind and a willingness to listen to your body, can unlock a world of profound physical, emotional, and mental benefits.

Myth #1:
Fasting is all about weight loss.

While the potential for weight management is often a primary motivator for individuals exploring intermittent fasting, the true benefits of this practice extend far beyond the scale. Through my own journey, I've come to understand that fasting is not just about shedding pounds, but about achieving a deeper sense of balance and harmony within the body.

Adapting to the rhythms of fasting, I noticed remarkable

changes in my overall well-being. My digestion improved, with fewer instances of bloating, acid reflux, and discomfort. My energy levels remained the same, and I found myself more alert and focused throughout the day. Perhaps most significantly, I slowly became more attuned to the subtle cues of my body and better able to discern the difference between true physical hunger and the constant need for immediate gratification.

You see, fasting isn't just about what we put into our bodies; it's also about what we take out - the constant barrage of stimuli, the emotional attachments to food, the subconscious patterns that have been driving our eating behaviors for years. By giving our digestive system a much-needed break, we create the space for deeper self-awareness, allowing us to uncover the root causes of our unhealthy relationships with food.

Myth #2: Fasting is an All-or-Nothing Approach.

Another common misconception about intermittent fasting is that it requires an extreme, rigid adherence to a specific set of rules. The belief that you must fast for extended periods, or that you can never deviate from a predetermined schedule, can be a significant barrier for those considering this practice.

However, as we'll explore in this section, the reality is far more nuanced and flexible. There is no one-size-fits-all approach, and the key is to find a personalized rhythm that aligns with your unique needs, preferences, and lifestyle.

As a lifestyle choice, intermittent fasting allows for flexibility and adjustments to suit your unique needs and circumstances. You make adjustments to it on the go. Let's say, as an example you have worked your fasting hours progressively and you don't usually have breakfast anymore. Then, it is your aunt's birthday and she invites all your family for breakfast. To eat or not to eat, that is the question. If you know in advance, you can probably shift your feeding window that day to allow for breakfast. Go to the party, have fun, enjoy life. Intermittent fasting is a process in which you learn to listen to your body, it should not be a restrictive regime like all the other diets.

For some, a simple 12-hour overnight fast may be the sweet spot, allowing their digestive system to complete its natural cycles without feeling overly deprived. For others, longer fasting windows of 16 or even 24 hours may be the path to greater well-being. And still, others may thrive on a more cyclical approach, alternating between periods of fasting and feasting depending on their energy levels, stress levels, and overall state of being.

The point is, fasting is not about perfection or adherence to a strict set of rules. It's about tuning in to the subtle cues of your body, experimenting with different approaches, and finding the rhythm that allows you to feel your best, both physically and mentally.

A 2018 review article published in Medical Clinics of North America by Drs. Kevin Hall and Scott Kahan[1] challenges the 'all or nothing' approach.

The researchers examined the complex factors that make long-term weight loss maintenance difficult, regardless of the dietary strategy employed. Hall and Kahan emphasize that weight regain is common due to a combination of biological, behavioral, and environmental influences that promote weight gain. They argue that no single approach, including intermittent fasting, necessitates perfect adherence to be effective in the long run. Instead, the authors stress the importance of flexibility, sustainability, and ongoing support for lasting success.

The review highlights the high degree of individual vari-

---

[1] Hall, Kevin D., and Scott Kahan. "Maintenance of Lost Weight and Long-Term Management of Obesity." Medical Clinics of North America 102, no. 1 (January 2018): 183–97. https://doi.org/10.1016/j.mcna.2017.08.012.

ability in weight loss maintenance within any given dietary intervention. This suggests that an 'all or nothing' mindset fails to account for personal differences and preferences. Hall and Kahan propose that the best approach is one that an individual can stick with over time.

Furthermore, the researchers underscore the persistent effort required to counteract the biological adaptations that drive weight regain. They contend that a short-term, rigid perspective on intermittent fasting is unlikely to yield enduring results. Rather, a long-term, adaptable approach is crucial.

This study provides a compelling evidence-based case against the 'all or nothing' myth surrounding intermittent fasting. It supports the idea that intermittent fasting can be a sustainable, effective tool for weight management when integrated into a healthy lifestyle with proper support and a long-term outlook.

Based on the information provided in the study, we can debunk the myth that "intermittent fasting is an all or nothing approach" in a few key ways:

1. The study highlights that long-term weight loss maintenance is very challenging, regardless of the dietary approach used. Weight regain is common due to complex

biological, behavioral, and environmental factors. This suggests that an "all or nothing" mentality is not realistic or necessary for any diet, including intermittent fasting. Flexibility and sustainability are key.

2. The authors recommend ongoing clinical support, counseling, and weight maintenance-specific strategies to improve long-term success. This implies that intermittent fasting does not have to be rigidly adhered to forever. Ongoing adjustments and support can help make it a sustainable part of a healthy lifestyle.

3. The study notes there is high individual variability in long-term weight loss success within any given dietary approach. Some may find intermittent fasting easier to stick with than others. An "all or nothing" view ignores these individual differences. The optimal approach is whichever one a person can maintain long-term.

4. Maintaining weight loss requires persistent effort over time to counter biological adaptations that promote weight regain. An "all or nothing" short-term mindset with intermittent fasting is unlikely to generate lasting results. The focus should be on long-term adherence.

In summary, this study on the science of long-term weight management supports the notion that intermittent fasting does not require perfect lifelong adherence to produce benefits. As with any approach, flexibility, individualization, and a long-term perspective are more important than an rigid "all or nothing" stance. Intermittent fasting can be a sustainable piece of a healthy lifestyle.

As you embark on this journey, I encourage you to approach it with a spirit of curiosity and self-compassion. Recognize that your relationship with food and your body is unique, and that the path to well-being may look different for you than it does for others. Be willing to try new things, to make adjustments, and to trust the wisdom of your own body.

Because at the end of the day, fasting is not about deprivation or restriction; it's about reclaiming your power, reconnecting with your true needs, and discovering the profound benefits that can arise when you approach your health and well-being with a holistic, mindful approach.

Myth #3
You will be hungry all the time.

One of my biggest fears was that I would be constantly plagued by hunger. I had always associated the idea of not eating with feelings of deprivation and discomfort. However, as I delved deeper into the research surrounding fasting, I came across a study that challenged this notion.

In 2010, Klempel and colleagues published a study in

the Nutrition Journal[2] that followed 16 obese adults on an alternate day fasting plan for 8 weeks. The participants limited their calorie intake to about 25% of their normal needs on "fast" days and ate freely on "feast" days. As I read through the study's findings, I was surprised to learn that while participants did report increased hunger in the first week or two, their hunger levels significantly decreased after about 2 weeks, even on fasting days.

Here's what they found: In the first week or two, participants did report increased hunger on fasting days. But after about 2 weeks, their hunger levels significantly decreased, even on days when they weren't eating much. Essentially, their bodies adapted to the new eating pattern and they stopped feeling so hungry on fasting days.

Not only did constant hunger fade away, but the participants actually started feeling more satisfied with the intermittent fasting diet after about a month. Although they never reported feeling "full" on fasting days, they weren't battling hunger all the time either.

The researchers think these findings mean intermittent fasting could be a sustainable long-term approach for

---

[2] Monica C. Klempel, Surabhi Bhutani, Marian Fitzgibbon, Sally Freels, and Krista A. Varady, "Dietary and Physical Activity Adaptations to Alternate Day Modified Fasting: Implications for Optimal Weight Loss," Nutrition Journal 9, no. 35 (2010), https://doi.org/10.1186/1475-2891-9-35

weight loss. The key is getting through those first couple of weeks. After that initial adjustment period, your body gets used to the routine and constant hunger shouldn't be an issue anymore.

So while you might feel hungrier at first when you start intermittent fasting, this study suggests that feeling is only temporary. After a few weeks, those hunger pangs should subside and you'll be more satisfied with your new eating habits. Don't let the myth of constant hunger stop you from giving intermittent fasting a try if you're interested in it for weight loss or other health benefits.

As you extend the duration of your fasts, you develop an understanding of your body's hunger. At first it is a ravenous all consuming force within you, then, slowly it becomes something more tame. It is one thing to consciously know that the human body can go without food for days, and another to wait to ingest food for another 2 hours. It sounds laughable, but the phrase "I'm starving" or "I'm dying of hunger" shouldn't be applicable for periods of time that can be counted in hours instead of days.

Myth #4
You can't focus while fasting.

When I first started intermittent fasting, I was concerned that the lack of food might leave me feeling foggy and unfocused. As someone who relies on mental clarity to tackle daily tasks and challenges, the idea of not being able to concentrate was a daunting prospect. However, as I dug deeper into the science behind fasting, I discovered that my fears may have been unfounded.

A detailed study published in the Annals of Medicine by Françoise Wilhelmi de Toledo and her team (2020)[3] shed light on how fasting affects our brain function. The researchers found that during fasting, our body starts producing ketones from fat, which serve as a kind of superfuel for the brain. This made me imagine ketones as a premium gasoline that helps a car run more efficiently, providing the brain with the energy it needs to perform at its best.

But the benefits didn't stop there. The study also revealed that fasting triggers the production of brain-derived neurotrophic factors (BDNF), a special protein that acts like a fertilizer for the brain. BDNF helps grow and strengthen brain cells, leading to better memory, learning, and overall brain health. This information was a game-changer for me, as it suggested that fasting could actually support my cognitive function, rather than hinder it.

As I continued to explore the world of intermittent fasting, I found that my personal experiences aligned with the study's findings. Despite my initial concerns, I discovered

---

[3] Wilhelmi de Toledo, Françoise, Franziska Grundler, Cesare R. Sirtori, and Massimiliano Ruscica. "Unravelling the Health Effects of Fasting: A Long Road from Obesity Treatment to Healthy Life Span Increase and Improved Cognition." Annals of Medicine 52, no. 5 (2020): 147-161. https://doi.org/10.1080/07853890.2020.1770849.

that on fasting days, I often felt a heightened sense of focus and mental clarity. It was as if the absence of food allowed my brain to operate more efficiently, tapping into the power of ketones and BDNF to keep me sharp and focused throughout the day.

A study by Jip Gudden and colleagues in the Nutrients journal (2021)[4] looked closely at how skipping meals at certain times (intermittent fasting) can help our brains work better. They found out that people who have trouble with memory or thinking clearly, including those with early Alzheimer's disease, showed improvement after they started fasting on and off. Basically, fasting helped their brains function better, making it easier for them to remember and think.

While the authors noted that short-term studies on healthy adults have shown inconsistent effects on cognition, they suggested this may be due to an initial adjustment period. As people regularly practice intermittent fasting, their bodies can adapt, potentially leading to improved focus and concentration.

The Gudden et al. review also highlighted animal studies that have demonstrated intermittent fasting can lead to

---

[4] Gudden, Jip, Alejandro Arias Vasquez, and Mirjam Bloemendaal. "The Effects of Intermittent Fasting on Brain and Cognitive Function." Nutrients 13, no. 9 (2021): 3166. https://doi.org/10.3390/nu13093166.

improved spatial memory, learning, and cognitive performance in various models of neurological disorders. This further supports the idea that fasting can actually support brain function, rather than impair it.

So, the evidence suggests that the common belief about not being able to focus while fasting may be a myth. The production of ketones and the upregulation of BDNF during fasting periods can provide the brain with an alternative fuel source and support cognitive function. While there may be an initial adjustment period, regular practice of intermittent fasting can help the body adapt, potentially leading to enhanced focus and concentration.

Myth #5
Fasting hinders muscle gain and accelerates muscle loss in older adults.

Have you ever heard that intermittent fasting hinders muscle gain or accelerates muscle loss, especially in older adults? It's a common myth that has been circulating in the health and wellness world for years. However, recent studies have provided evidence that intermittent fasting can be beneficial for both muscle gain in resistance-trained individuals and muscle maintenance in gracefully aging adults.

For those engaged in resistance training, a study by Tinsley and colleagues (2019)[5] found that intermittent fasting does not hinder muscle growth or performance improvements when combined with a proper exercise program and adequate calorie and protein intake. This means that individuals can enjoy the benefits of fasting while still making gains in the gym.

In the study, researchers compared the effects of time-restricted feeding (TRF) to a normal eating schedule (control diet, CD) in a group of resistance-trained women over an 8-week period. The TRF group ate all of their daily calories within a 7.5-hour window, while the CD group ate throughout the day. Both groups followed the same resistance training program and consumed similar amounts of calories and protein.

After 8 weeks, the researchers found that both the TRF and CD groups experienced similar increases in fat-free mass (which includes muscle mass), muscle thickness in

---

5 Tinsley, Grant M., M. Lane Moore, Austin J. Graybeal, Antonio Paoli, Youngdeok Kim, Joaquin U. Gonzales, John R. Harry, Trisha A. VanDusseldorp, Devin N. Kennedy, and Megan R. Cruz. "Time-Restricted Feeding Plus Resistance Training in Active Females: A Randomized Trial." The American Journal of Clinical Nutrition 110, no. 3 (2019): 628-640. https://doi.org/10.1093/ajcn/nqz126.

the arms and legs, and improvements in strength and endurance. These findings suggest that intermittent fasting does not hinder muscle growth or performance improvements when combined with resistance training.

3
Listening To Our Bodies

As I imagined the flickering flames cast a warm glow over the tribe's gathering, I couldn't help but be transported back in time - back to the world of my hunter-gatherer ancestors, where the rhythms of feast and famine were not just a physical reality, but a way of being. In their lives, the ebb and flow of abundance and scarcity was not a source of deprivation, but a dance of adaptation and resilience - a dance that held the keys to their very survival.

Imagine the erratic nature of food availability that these early humans faced. Unlike the constant, ever-present supply that we enjoy in the modern world, their sustenance was subject to the whims of the natural world - the migrations of the animals, the blooming and withering of the plants, the unpredictable tides of the seasons.

During times of plenty, when the hunt was successful or the foraging bountiful, they would feast, their bodies eagerly absorbing the nourishment they had so hard-won. In those moments they would readily store excess energy as fat - a survival mechanism that ensured they had a reserve to draw upon when the lean times came.

Our hunter-gatherer ancestors understood, on the deepest level, that their very existence was inextricably linked to the rhythms of the natural world. When the animals moved on and the plants withered, leaving them facing the prospect of going without sustenance for days, perhaps even weeks, they would draw upon the wisdom of their ancestors.

Through a process of metabolic adaptation, their metabolism would slow, their bodies becoming more efficient in their use of those precious calories. And as their hunger pangs subsided, they would find themselves imbued with a newfound clarity, their senses heightened, their focus sharpened. It was as if the very act of fasting had unlocked a wellspring of vitality within them – a wellspring that had been there all along, waiting to be tapped.

But this metabolic shift was not just about physical survival - it also had profound implications for their mental and emotional well-being. You see, during these periods of fasting, their bodies would enter a state of ketosis[1], where fat was broken down into ketones to fuel the brain and other vital organs. This process not only provided a steady, reliable source of energy, but also triggered a cascade of beneficial effects, including enhanced cognitive function, improved mood, and even the activation of a process called autophagy.

Autophagy, a term derived from the Greek words "auto" (self) and "phagy" (to eat), is a cellular process in which damaged or dysfunctional components are broken down and recycled. This process is particularly important during times of stress or nutrient deprivation, as it allows the body to conserve resources and clear out any harmful or unnecessary materials. For our hunter-gatherer ancestors, the act of fasting was a natural trigger for this process, helping to maintain the delicate balance of their bodies and minds.

Embracing the practice of intermittent fasting and mimicking the rhythms of feast and famine, I've been struck by the profound parallels between my own experience and the lives of my ancestors. I've felt the ebb and flow of my energy, the subtle shifts in my mental clarity, and

---

1 The Nutrition Source. 'Diet Review: Ketogenic Diet for Weight Loss.' Harvard T.H. Chan School of Public Health, accessed April 10, 2024. https://www.hsph.harvard.edu/nutritionsource/healthy-weight/diet-reviews/ketogenic-diet/

the way my body seems to hum with a newfound vitality when honoring its natural cycles.

For you see, the truth is that our bodies and minds are still wired to the rhythms of a bygone era – an era where the ebb and flow of feast and famine was not just a reality, but a way of being. In a world that has become so deeply disconnected from the natural world, the act of embracing these ancient cycles can serve as a powerful antidote to the health challenges that have become all too common in our contemporary societies.

Consider the scourge of obesity and type 2 diabetes that has gripped so many societies in the developed world. These are conditions that were virtually unknown to our foraging forebears, whose bodies were primed to thrive in the face of the natural cycles of abundance and scarcity.

In the wake of the Agricultural Revolution and the subsequent industrialization of our food systems, we have found ourselves trapped in a vicious cycle of constant consumption and metabolic dysfunction. Our bodies, still wired to the survival mechanisms of our ancestral past, have struggled to adapt to the relentless onslaught of processed, calorie-dense foods – a mismatch that has led to a host of chronic health issues.

But what if we could reclaim the wisdom of our hunter-gatherer ancestors? What if, by embracing the rhythms of intermittent fasting and the ebb and flow of feast and famine, we could unlock the keys to a more resilient, adaptable, and vibrant way of being?

That's precisely the journey that I've been on, and the results have been nothing short of transformative. As I've incorporated various intermittent fasting methods into my life – from the 16/8 time-restricted eating protocol to the occasional 24-hour fast – I've been amazed by the profound impact it has had on my physical, mental, and emotional well-being.

Gone are the constant struggles with bloating, acid reflux, and digestive discomfort that had plagued me for years. In their place, I've experienced a newfound clarity of mind, a surge of energy, and a deeper sense of connection to the natural rhythms that govern my existence. It's as if, by honoring the cyclical nature of my hunger and nourishment, I've unlocked a wellspring of vitality that had been there all along, waiting to be tapped.

The benefits extend far beyond the physical realm. I've found myself drawn into a deeper state of self-reflection, a space where I can explore the emotional and psychological factors that have shaped my relationship with food over the years. It's a process of self-discovery that has been both humbling and empowering, as I've peeled back the layers of my conditioning and reconnected with the innate wisdom of my body.

The truth is that the keys to our health and happiness have been there all along, encoded into our being. We are the descendants of a lineage that knew how to thrive in the face of adversity, to adapt to the ever-changing tides of the natural world. By tapping into that primal rhythm, by honoring the cycles of feast and famine that have guided our species for millennia, we just might unlock the secrets to a more harmonious, fulfilling way of living.

Of course, the journey of integrating this ancient wisdom into our modern lives is not without its challenges. We are, after all, the products of a society that has become accustomed to the constant availability of food, where the temptation to indulge our cravings is ever-present and the social pressures to conform can be overwhelming.

But as we peel back the layers of our conditioning and reclaim our innate connection to the natural world, we may just find that the true obstacles we face are not external, but internal – the deeply ingrained habits, the emotional attachments, the fears and anxieties that have kept us trapped in a cycle of unhealthy relationships with food.

And it is here, in the quiet moments of self-reflection and introspection, that the lessons of our hunter-gatherer ancestors can truly shine. For they knew, in the deepest recesses of their being, that the path to true nourishment and well-being was not about rigid adherence to rules or the pursuit of perfection, but about a deep, abiding respect for the natural rhythms that govern our world.

So, as we navigate the challenges of integrating this ancient wisdom into our contemporary lives, let us approach the journey with the same spirit of curiosity, resilience, and adaptability that our forebears embodied. Let us be willing to experiment, to make mistakes, to listen deeply to the whispers of our bodies and the wisdom of our hearts.

For in doing so, we just might uncover the secret to a more harmonious, fulfilling way of living – one that is rooted in the timeless rhythms of our ancestral past, yet perfectly suited to the demands of the present. A way of being that honors the ebb and flow of our hunger, the cycles of our energy, the innate intelligence that courses through our veins.

It is a path that is not always easy, but one that holds the promise of profound transformation. As we walk it together, drawing strength from the wisdom of our ancestors and the insights of our own lived experience, we may just find that the true nourishment we seek lies not in the endless pursuit of food, but in the deep, abiding connection to the rhythms that sustain us all.

Connecting Ancient Rhythms to Intermittent Fasting

Consider the concept of time-restricted eating, where individuals cycle between periods of fasting and feeding throughout the day. This method closely mimics the natural rhythms of our ancestral past, where food wasn't always readily available, and eating was often limited to specific times when sustenance was abundant.

In the hunter-gatherer lifestyle, the natural pattern was to forage and hunt during the daylight hours, fueling the body with the nourishment it needed to thrive. But as the sun dipped below the horizon, the tribe would transition into a state of rest and restoration, allowing their digestive systems a much-needed break from the constant influx of food.

It's a rhythm that is deeply ingrained in our biology – a legacy of our evolutionary past that, when honored, can have profound implications for our health and well-being. For just as our ancestors' bodies adapted to the cycles of feast and famine, so too can our own metabolisms become more efficient and resilient when we create intentional periods of fasting.

The benefits extend far beyond the physical realm. When the body is not constantly occupied with the process of digestion, it can free up mental and emotional resources that allow for more introspection and self-awareness. We create the space for deeper self-reflection, for the cultivation of patience and discipline, for the rediscovery of our deep, primal connection to the natural world.

It's a lesson that we can see echoed in other intermittent fasting methods as well. Take, for instance, the practice of alternate-day fasting, where individuals alternate between days of normal eating and days of minimal calorie intake. This rhythm could be seen as a structured adaptation of the unpredictable feast and famine periods experienced by our hunter-gatherer ancestors, where a successful hunt or foraging expedition would be followed by days without such abundance.

Or consider the 5:2 diet, which involves eating normally for five days of the week and restricting calorie intake to 500-600 calories on the other two days. This method can be viewed as a nod to the occasional scarcity of food that would have forced our ancestors to go through periods of reduced intake, interspersed with days of normal or increased eating when sustenance was plentiful.

And then there's the Eat-Stop-Eat approach, which involves a 24-hour fast once or twice a week, with normal eating during the rest of the time. This method directly mirrors the involuntary fasting that our hunter-gatherer forebears would have experienced regularly, due to unsuccessful hunts or the lack of available forage.

Each of these fasting methods, in its own way, reflects the natural eating patterns of our ancestors – patterns that were driven not by the pursuit of weight loss or the latest health fad, but by the simple, primal necessity of survival. By incorporating these practices into our modern lives, we have the opportunity to not only reap the physical benefits, but to also reconnect with the timeless wisdom that has been passed down through the generations.

The Hunter-Gatherer Diet: Nourishing the Body, Nurturing the Soul

Early human's relationship with food was not merely a matter of survival, but a profound expression of their deep, innate connection to the natural world. For in the rhythms of feast and famine, they had discovered a wisdom that extended far beyond the physical plane, touching upon the very essence of what it means to be human.

Consider the diversity of their diet. Where we in the modern age have become accustomed to the monotony of a few staple crops – wheat, rice, maize – our foraging forebears feasted on a wide variety of natural foods. From the succulent fruits of the forest to the lean, protein-rich meats of the hunt, their plates featured a diverse array of flavors, textures, and nutritional riches. As Yuval Noah Harari notes in his book "Sapiens: A Brief History of Humankind," the diet of hunter-gatherers was not only remarkably varied compared to many humans today, but also generally well-balanced, providing a wide range of essential nutrients.[2]

And it was not just the sheer variety of their sustenance that set them apart, but the way in which they approached the act of nourishment itself. For these were people who understood, on the deepest level, that true well-being was not just about filling the belly, but about honoring the intricate web of life that sustained them.

They knew, for instance, that the act of hunting was not

---

[2] Harari, Yuval N. Sapiens: A Brief History of Humankind. New York: Harper, 2014.

merely a means to an end, but a sacred ritual imbued with reverence and respect. When they tracked and felled their prey, they did so with a deep awareness of the animal's role in the ecosystem, offering a prayer of gratitude for the sustenance it would provide. And in the preparation and consumption of their food, they engaged in a dance of mindfulness, savoring each bite and allowing the flavors to transport them to the very heart of the natural world.

It was a way of living that was, in many ways, the antithesis of the frenetic, disconnected existence that has become the norm in our modern societies. For where we so often find ourselves caught in the endless cycle of mindless consumption, our hunter-gatherer ancestors had cultivated a profound sense of presence and connection – a way of being that allowed them to truly nourish not just their bodies, but their souls.

As I contemplate the lessons of their past, I've come to realize that this wisdom is not just a relic of a bygone era, but a wellspring of insight that holds the potential to transform our own lives in profound and lasting ways.

For in the diversity of the hunter-gatherer diet, we find a blueprint for true holistic health – a way of eating that nourishes not just our physical bodies, but the intricate web of our emotional, mental, and spiritual well-being. By embracing a wider range of whole, unprocessed foods – the vibrant greens, the nutrient-dense roots, the succulent proteins – we can begin to reclaim the vitality and balance that our ancestors so effortlessly embodied.

Furthermore, in the ritual and reverence with which they approached the act of nourishment, we discover a path to a more mindful, present, and fulfilling relationship with food. For it is in the slowing down, the savoring, the deep appreciation for the gifts of the natural world, that we can begin to transcend the endless cycle of mindless consumption and rediscover the true joy and sustenance that food can provide.

It's about rediscovering the joy of preparing meals from scratch, of savoring the unique flavors and textures of whole, unprocessed ingredients. It's about cultivating a deep appreciation for the seasonal rhythms that govern the availability of different foods, and allowing those cycles to guide our own patterns of consumption.

Perhaps most importantly, it's about reconnecting with the innate wisdom of our bodies – learning to discern the difference between true physical hunger and the constant cravings that so often drive us to overindulge. It's about embracing the ebb and flow of our energy levels, honoring the natural rhythms that govern our sleep, our activity, and our need for rest and restoration.

In doing so, we may just find that the true nourishment we seek is not just about what we put into our bodies, but about the way we approach the entire process of sustaining ourselves. It's about reclaiming the reverence, the ritual, and the deep, abiding connection to the natural world that was once the birthright of our hunter-gatherer ancestors.

4
Emotional Hunger Vs. Physical Hunger

As we've explored the primal rhythms of feast and famine that once governed the lives of our hunter-gatherer ancestors, we've uncovered a profound truth - that the gnawing, all-consuming signals we associate with hunger are not just about the physical need for nourishment, but are inextricably bound to the complex emotional landscape that shapes our relationship with food.

In the previous chapter, we delved into the evolutionary wisdom inherent in these ancient cycles, and how embracing the ebb and flow of sustenance can unlock a wellspring of vitality, resilience, and self-awareness. It's become increasingly clear that the true challenge lies not just in mastering the physical act of fasting, but in untangling the tangled web of emotions, habits, and psychological conditioning that have long held our approach to nourishment in their grip.

In this chapter, we'll explore the complex interplay between our physical and emotional needs, and how recognizing the distinction between the two can unlock a deeper level of self-awareness and empowerment. We'll touch upon the concept of "hanger" - that all-too-familiar sensation of a rumbling, hollow stomach, a prickly irritability, and a sense of distress that can arise when our hunger goes unmet - and examine the latest research on the psychological mechanisms that underlie this phenomenon.

Most importantly, we'll equip you with practical tools and strategies for differentiating between the gnawing ache of physical hunger and the intense, often insatiable craving that springs from the wellspring of our emotions. By cultivating this heightened level of internal perception awareness - this keen sensitivity to the subtle cues of our bodies and minds - you'll not only find greater success in your fasting practice, but also unlock a newfound sense of balance, resilience, and overall well-being.

So, let us take a closer look, armed with open hearts and curious minds. For in unraveling the secrets that lie beneath the surface of our hunger, we may just uncover the keys to a more vibrant, balanced, and joyful way of living.

Defining Hunger and Its Bodily Sensations

At its core, hunger is a biological signal that our bodies use to communicate a need for nourishment. When our energy reserves start to dwindle, our brains and bodies respond by triggering a cascade of physiological changes - a rumbling, hollow sensation in the pit of the stomach, a feeling of emptiness that seems to expand and contract with each passing minute, an increased desire to seek out and consume food. These are the visceral, embodied cues that motivate us to seek sustenance and restore the balance our bodies crave.

The study "The Development of Interoceptive Hunger Signals"[1] has revealed that these internal hunger cues are not innate or hardwired responses, it's important to note that the specific sensations we associate with hunger can

---

1 Stevenson, R. J., Bartlett, J., Wright, M., Hughes, A., Hill, B. J., Saluja, S., & Francis, H. M. (2023). The development of interoceptive hunger signals. Developmental Psychobiology, 65, e22374. https://doi.org/10.1002/dev.22374

vary significantly from individual to individual. This is because our perception and interpretation of hunger signals are heavily influenced by our early life experiences and the cues and behaviors modeled by our primary caregivers.

For some, the experience of hunger may be marked by a distinct, rumbling sensation in the stomach, while for others, it may manifest as a feeling of fatigue or nausea. These variations in how we interpret and respond to hunger cues are a clear indication of the highly personal and subjective nature of this phenomenon. By recognizing that our hunger sensations are not universally felt, but rather shaped by our unique histories and learned associations, we can develop a deeper understanding and compassion for the diverse ways in which hunger is experienced.

The Concept of "Hangry" and Its Effects on Emotions

One of the most widely recognized phenomena related to hunger is the concept of "hangry" - the experience of becoming irritable, short-tempered, or emotionally dysregulated when our hunger goes unmet. This phenomenon has been the subject of extensive research, and the findings shed important light on the intricate relationship between our physical and emotional states.

A study published in the APA Journal Emotion "Feeling Hangry? When Hunger Is Conceptualized as Emotion"[2] delved into the psychological mechanisms behind the "hangry" experience. The researchers found that when we're hungry, our brains tend to interpret the physical sensations of hunger through the lens of our emotional state, often perceiving them as a threat or source of distress. This is because the brain regions responsible for processing hunger and emotion are closely interconnected, with the amygdala - the part of the brain that regulates our emotional responses - playing a key role in how we interpret and respond to hunger cues.

When our bodies signal a need for food, the amygdala can interpret this as a potential threat to our well-being, triggering a cascade of physiological and emotional responses, including increased irritability, anxiety, and even aggression. It's as if the rumbling in our stomachs and the fatigue in our limbs become inextricably linked to feelings of frustration, anger, and a sense of unease that can color our entire outlook on the world around us.

The amygdala's reaction to hunger signals serves an important evolutionary purpose. When the body senses a

---

[2] MacCormack, Jennifer K., and Kristen A. Lindquist. "Feeling Hangry? When Hunger Is Conceptualized as Emotion." Emotion 19, no. 2 (2019): 301-319. https://doi.org/10.1037/emo0000422

lack of nourishment, the amygdala interprets this as a potential threat to survival. This "hangry" state likely evolved as a way to motivate our ancestors to seek out food and ensure their survival during times of scarcity. Understanding the amygdala's role in this process can help us recognize and manage our emotional responses to hunger more effectively.

Is Being "Hangry" Real or Imagined?

Given the subjective nature of the "hangry" experience, it's natural to wonder whether it's a real, measurable phenomenon or simply a figment of our imagination. After all, we've all had moments where we've blamed our irritability or short-temper on hunger, only to realize that the problem may have been more emotional than physical.

However, a study published in the Journal PLOS ONE "Hangry in the Field: An Experience Sampling Study on the Impact of Hunger on Anger, Irritability, and Affect"[3] provides compelling evidence that the "hangry" experience is indeed a tangible and measurable reality. In this study, researchers used an experience sampling method to track the real-time emotional and physiological states of participants as they went about their daily lives. They

---

[3] Swami V, Hochstoger S, Kargl E, Stieger S (2022) Hangry in the field: An experience sampling study on the impact of hunger on anger, irritability, and affect. PLoS ONE 17(7): e0269629.https://doi.org/10.1371/journal.pone.0269629

found that when participants reported feeling hungry, they also exhibited significantly higher levels of anger, irritability, and negative affect, compared to when they were not experiencing hunger.

Importantly, these emotional changes were not simply a matter of subjective perception - the researchers also observed corresponding physiological changes, such as increased heart rate and skin conductance, that are associated with the experience of negative emotions. It's as if the very act of our bodies signaling a need for nourishment triggers a cascade of physiological and psychological responses that can profoundly shape our mood and our behavior.

A Mindful Approach to Breaking Hunger-Related Habits

It's become clear that the key to navigating this landscape lies in cultivating a greater sense of self-awareness and mindfulness. By learning to recognize the subtle differences between emotional and physical hunger, we can begin to break free from the habitual patterns and knee-jerk reactions that so often govern our relationship with food.

In a powerful TED Talk, psychiatrist and neuroscientist

Judson Brewer[4] shared insights on how a curious, awareness-based approach can be applied to breaking deeply ingrained habits, including those related to eating and hunger. As I sat mesmerized by his words, I couldn't help but reflect on the profound impact this mindful perspective could have on navigating the complex landscape of emotional and physical hunger.

Brewer explained that the key lies in developing a heightened sense of interoceptive awareness - the ability to tune in to the subtle physical and emotional cues that arise within our bodies. When it comes to hunger, this means paying close attention to the specific sensations and feelings that arise when we experience the urge to eat. Is it a rumbling in the stomach, a sense of fatigue, or a craving for a particular food? Or is it a feeling of restlessness, irritability, or a desire for comfort or distraction?

By becoming more attuned to these nuanced differences, we can start to recognize the patterns and triggers that underlie our hunger-related behaviors. And rather than simply acting on these impulses, we can pause, observe, and consciously choose how to respond. This heightened level of self-awareness allows us to break free from the cycle of mindless consumption and instead, approach

---

4 Brewer, Judson. "A Simple Way to Break a Bad Habit." TED Talks. February 2016. https://www.ted.com/talks/judson_brewer_a_simple_way_to_break_a_bad_habit/transcript?language=en&subtitle=en

nourishment with intention, balance, and a deep understanding of our true needs.

Judson Brewer's insights struck a deep chord within me. He spoke of how a mindful, curious approach could be the key to unraveling even our most entrenched habits - the ones that seem to have a vice-like grip on our bodies and minds.

Brewer explained that the secret lies in tuning into the subtle physical and emotional sensations that arise when we experience the urge to engage in these habitual behaviors. Rather than trying to forcefully resist the craving, he suggested we become intimate explorers of its very nature. What does the restlessness feel like in my belly? How does the irritability prickle along my skin? Is there a faint yearning, a whisper of comfort or distraction, underlying the impulse?

To uncover these patterns, Brewer encouraged keeping a detailed food and mood journal - a practice that would allow me to shed light on the specific cues, be they environmental, hormonal or psychological, that tend to activate my hunger-driven habits. Perhaps it's the familiar pull towards the vending machine when the afternoon slump hits, or the urge to mindlessly snack while watching TV in the evenings. But the real power lies in not just observing these triggers, but in cultivating the ability to separate myself from the sensations themselves.

Rather than simply identifying with the craving as an extension of who I am, I could learn to become the impartial observer, noticing the physical and emotional experiences as they arise, without judgment. Is this sensation a fleeting discomfort that will pass, or a deeper need for nourishment, rest or emotional fulfillment? By approaching hunger with this mindful curiosity and self-awareness, I would have the opportunity to pause, observe, and consciously choose how to respond - to give in to the temptation or to weather it out and see what happens. In that moment of clarity we can break free from the cycle of mindless consumption and instead, cultivate a balanced, intentional relationship with food.

Emotional Hunger vs. Physical Hunger

At the heart of the distinction between emotional and physical hunger lies the fundamental difference between desire and necessity. Physical hunger is a biological imperative - a genuine need for nourishment that our bodies communicate through a variety of sensory cues. It's the feeling of an empty, rumbling stomach, a lack of energy, or a sense of physical discomfort that drives us to seek out food.

Emotional hunger, on the other hand, is rooted in psychological and emotional factors, rather than physical need. It's the craving for comfort, distraction, or a sense of pleasure or reward that leads us to seek out food, even when our bodies are not truly in need of sustenance. This type of hunger is often characterized by an intense, almost insatiable desire for a specific food or indulgence, rather than a general need for nourishment.

Differentiating Between Emotional and Physical Hunger

So, how can we distinguish between emotional and physical hunger?[5] Here are four key ways to recognize the difference:

1. **Timing and Intensity:** Physical hunger announces itself gradually; it's a creeping sensation of emptiness that slowly intensifies, signaling the body's genuine need for sustenance. Imagine the gentle build-up from a whisper of "I might need to eat soon" to a decisive "It's definitely time to eat." This type of hunger is patient, giving you time to respond thoughtfully. In stark contrast, emotional hunger strikes swiftly and with force. It's the sudden,

---

[5] Clegg, Jennifer. "Four Easy, Effective Ways to Distinguish Emotional Hunger." LinkedIn. Accessed April, 10 2024. https://www.linkedin.com/pulse/four-easy-effective-ways-distinguish-emotional-hunger-clegg-lpc/

compelling urge to eat that can ambush you in moments of stress or boredom—like that intense craving for a snack when you're stuck in traffic, frustration mounting by the minute. This hunger is impulsive and urgent, demanding immediate satisfaction and often leaving you with a lingering sense of guilt.

2. **Specific Cravings**: Physical hunger is an open invitation from your body, calling for any type of nourishment without particular preferences; it is a general call for sustenance. This type of hunger is accommodating, suggesting that you could eat just about anything to satisfy the body's basic needs. Conversely, emotional hunger is selective and precise. It often manifests as an intense craving for a specific type of comfort food or treat, like suddenly needing a Snickers bar when you're feeling down or stressed. This isn't merely hunger—it's a specific demand driven by your emotions, seeking a particular flavor or experience as a form of solace or reward. Unlike the broad spectrum of physical hunger, emotional hunger zeroes in on exact items, often those linked to comfort or nostalgia.

3. **Satisfaction and Satiety:** When we eat in response to physical hunger, we tend to feel a sense of satisfaction and fullness once we've consumed an appropriate amount of food. Emotional hunger, on the other hand, is often insatiable, with the desire to keep eating even after

we've met our physical needs.

4. **Emotional Triggers:** Emotional hunger often manifests above the neck—it is an idea, a sudden thought provoked by emotions like stress, boredom, or the pursuit of comfort. You might find yourself salivating at the sight of a decadent dessert, driven not by an empty stomach but by a craving stimulated by your mood or thoughts. Physical hunger, in contrast, is experienced below the neck. It originates in your gut, a straightforward, biological signal from your body that it requires fuel. This type of hunger builds gradually, marked by a stomach rumble or, in prolonged cases, perhaps even a headache, indicating that your physical need for food has become urgent.

The true key to navigating the fasting journey lies not just in mastering the technical aspects of intermittent fasting, but in cultivating a deeper level of self-awareness and emotional intelligence. By learning to distinguish between the physical sensations of hunger and the emotional triggers that can drive our cravings and behaviors, we unlock a powerful pathway to greater balance, resilience, and overall well-being.

We can begin to break free from the habitual patterns and knee-jerk reactions that have so often governed our relationship with food, and instead, approach nourishment with a greater sense of mindfulness, intention, and self-compassion.

As we close this chapter, I can't help but feel a sense of both excitement and trepidation. The insights we've uncovered about the complex interplay between our physical and emotional hunger have cracked open a window into a whole new realm of self-understanding. But the prospect of truly reckoning with these patterns - of facing them head-on with curiosity rather than avoidance - can feel like trudging through the fires of hell.

Still, as Winston Churchill once said, 'If you're going through hell, keep going.' So that is what we must do. No more hemming and hawing, no more making excuses. Instead, let's approach this journey of self-discovery with the unflinching resolve of a seasoned explorer. Armed with the practical tools and strategies we've gathered, let's dive in, ready to observe our hunger cravings with a scientist's detachment and a seeker's wonder.

Because I believe that in doing so - in truly getting to know the rhythms and contours of our own experience - we just might uncover the keys to a more balanced, intentional relationship with food. It won't be easy, and there will undoubtedly be setbacks along the way. But if we can learn to view our hunger not as an enemy to be conquered, but as a teacher to be listened to, we may emerge from this process with a profound sense of self-awareness and the capacity to nourish ourselves, body and soul.

5
Fueling Your Fasted Workouts

As we explored in the previous chapter, fasting has the power to unlock profound benefits, both physical and mental. Central to these benefits is the body's ability to shift between utilizing glucose and fat as its primary fuel sources. This metabolic flexibility - the capacity to choreograph a dance between these two energy sources - is something our bodies are designed to do, but it's a skill that often needs to be relearned and refined through consistent fasting practice.

Typically, our bodies rely primarily on glucose, derived from the carbohydrates in our diet, as their main source of fuel. However, when we enter a fasted state and deplete our readily available glucose stores, our metabolism begins to adapt, transitioning to break down stored fat into ketones that can then be used as an alternative energy source. This process of switching between glucose-burning and fat-burning, known as ketosis, takes time and consistency to fully master, but the benefits can be profound.

I've personally experienced this transition from a glucose-burning to a fat-adapted state, it carries both challenges and rewards. In the beginning, I did feel a bit sluggish, as if I had walked for hours on end, as my body adjusted to utilizing fat as its primary fuel source. But with patience and consistency, I began to notice a remarkable shift in my energy levels and overall physical performance. But the real challenge was the internal battle raging in my mind.

On one hand, I found myself constantly preoccupied with thoughts of food, craving the comfort and familiarity of my old eating habits. There was a part of me that just wanted to give in, to abandon this experiment and return to the complacency of my previous routines.

Yet, on the other hand, I felt a growing sense of pride and accomplishment each time I completed a fasting window. It was as if I was unlocking a new level of discipline and self-awareness, my mind infused with a clarity I hadn't experienced in years. The hunger pangs gradually subsided, and I began to notice a remarkable shift in my energy and mental focus during my fasts.

With time and consistent practice, the sluggishness gave way to a sense of increased vitality and efficiency. It was as if my body had been given a tune-up, operating with a newfound power and precision. No longer was I bogged down by the constant need for glucose – instead, I felt a steady, reliable source of energy coursing through me, fueled by the fat stores my body had learned to tap into.

With my body becoming more adept at switching between glucose and fat as primary fuel sources, I was eager to see how this metabolic flexibility would impact my physical performance. After all, if my body was becoming more efficient at tapping into its fat stores for energy, I wondered how that might translate to my workouts and exercise routines.

You see, I've always enjoyed being active and moving my body, though I've never considered myself a high-performing athlete. As a kid, I swam competitively and later took up karate in my teens. In my 20s, I played a lot of squash, and over the years, I've incorporated running into my exercise routine as well. It's never been my priority to push the limits or compete at an elite level - I'm simply someone who genuinely derives joy and fulfillment from being physically active.

So as I continued on this journey of intermittent fasting and fat-adaptation, I was curious to see how it might impact the way I approached my workouts and other physical activities. Would I notice a difference in my energy levels, my endurance, or even my mental focus during exercise? And more importantly, would these changes align with my own personal fitness goals and the way I like to engage with movement?

At first, I'll admit, my brain did play a bit of a trick on me. Even though I knew my body was now better equipped to utilize fat for fuel, that old mental conditioning still tried to hold me back. After not having eaten for hours, far more than what I was accustomed to, I had this nagging feeling that I needed to go easy on myself, that I needed to work out at a lower intensity. Which was understandable, but as I came to realize, my mind had its own sneaky ways of trying to hold me back.

Now, I know it can feel a bit complex to wrap your head around the differences between burning glucose versus fat for fuel. But let me tell you, it's a lot like that classic children's tale, "The Little Train That Could." Remember that determined little locomotive, chugging its way up the hill, pulling all those heavy cars? That's kind of how I felt at first.

"Oh, I haven't eaten in so long. Can I really pull this off? Is the workload too heavy?" But you know what? Just like that plucky little train, I was surprised by what my body was capable of. Don't be a victim of your own mind - just put one foot in front of the other and see what happens. You may just amaze yourself.

The reality is, working out in a fasted state does feel a bit different in the body. Part of it is because you are utilizing a different fuel source - ketones instead of glucose. But another key factor is the way your mind tries to convince you that you ought to reduce your effort, that you're not capable of your usual intensity or performance.

This metabolic flexibility took hold and my body became more adept at switching between glucose and fat as primary fuel sources, I was eager to see how it would impact my physical performance. After all, if my body was becoming more efficient at tapping into its fat stores for energy, I wondered how that might translate to my workouts and exercise routines.

To further explore this concept, I turned to a study published in the Journal of Applied Physiology[1], which provided some fascinating insights. The researchers found that people who trained in a fasted state, without eating beforehand, showed greater benefits when it came to exercise capacity and endurance.

In layman's terms, the key takeaways were that training on an empty stomach led to more effective use of fat stores for energy during exercise. This meant the body became better at tapping into those fat reserves, which could be particularly beneficial for endurance activities like running or cycling. Additionally, those who trained fasted were better able to maintain stable blood sugar levels, which is crucial for avoiding energy dips and supporting the recovery process.

Working out at the beginning of my fasted state, 1 or 2 hours after eating, feels different compared to the end of my fasted window, 16 hours since my last meal. In the early stages of my fast, I find that my body responds better to more explosive, high-intensity interval workouts. The quick, readily available energy from carbohydrates allows for a sense of rapid response and explosive power.

---

[1] Van Proeyen, Karen, Karolina Szlufcik, Henri Nielens, Monique Ramaekers, and Peter Hespel. "Beneficial Metabolic Adaptations Due to Endurance Exercise Training in the Fasted State." Journal of Applied Physiology 110, no. 1 (2011): 236-245. Accessed [April 2024]. https://www.ncbi.nlm.nih.gov/pmc/articles/PMC3253005

However, as I progress deeper into my fasted state, I've come to appreciate the unique benefits of exercising in a fat-adapted, ketone-fueled state. My body has learned to efficiently tap into its fat reserves, providing a steadier, more sustainable source of fuel. This translates to a different kind of energy - one that may feel more even-keeled, without the sharp peaks and valleys. And crucially, my body is less reliant on that finite glycogen supply, allowing me to maintain my effort for longer periods of time.

The reason I prefer to time my more intense workouts towards the end of my fasting window is that my next meal is near, and my body will soon have the opportunity to replenish its reserves. By exercising in this fat-adapted state, I'm able to push myself harder and for longer, knowing that I'll be able to refuel and recover effectively once I break my fast

I've found that for activities like medium to long-distance running, the end of my fasted state is my preferred time to exercise. My mind feels clear, focused, and I can lose myself in my thoughts and the rhythm of my movement, almost effortlessly. It's as if my body and my brain have been given a tune-up, operating with newfound precision and efficiency.

Of course, as with any new approach to exercise and nutrition, it's important to listen to your body and make adjustments as needed. What works for me may not be the perfect fit for you. The key is to experiment, to be patient and compassionate with yourself, and to trust the process as your body adapts and finds its own unique rhythm.

Don't just take my word for it, though. Give it a good 1 to 3 months, and see for yourself. I'm not an elite athlete, by any means - just a regular person who enjoys moving my body and having fun. And let me tell you, the mental clarity I've gained has been a game-changer.

As I look back on the journey that has brought me to this point, I'm filled with a deep sense of gratitude and wonder. Who would have thought that by simply allowing my body to rest and reset, I would unlock such profound physical and mental benefits? It's as if I've been gifted a new lease on life, my energy, endurance, and cognitive functions all operating at a higher level than I ever imagined possible.

I encourage you to keep that little train chugging forward, to trust in the wisdom of your body and the power of your own determination. For in doing so, you just might surprise yourself with the incredible heights you're able to reach. The rewards, both physical and mental, are there for the taking - all you have to do is take that first step.

Integrating fasting with your workout regimen isn't just about physical endurance—it's about retraining and optimizing your body's energy use for a healthier, more vibrant life. Fasting enhances metabolic flexibility, allowing your body to efficiently switch from using glucose to burning fat. This transition not only boosts physical performance but also sharpens mental clarity.

You've learned about the initial challenges of adapting to a fasted state, such as feeling sluggish or battling cravings, and how consistency and patience play crucial roles in overcoming these hurdles. By persisting through these early difficulties, you can unlock a new level of energy efficiency and endurance that extends beyond the gym to every part of your daily life.

I encourage you to view fasting and exercise not as a short-term diet or fitness trend but as a sustainable lifestyle change. It offers profound benefits that go beyond simple weight loss, providing enhanced cognitive function and a greater sense of overall well-being. As you begin or continue your journey with fasting workouts, remember to listen to your body, adjust your routines as necessary, and most importantly, trust the process.

The path to discovering your body's full potential is not

without its challenges, but the rewards of enhanced energy, endurance, and mental clarity are well worth the effort. Keep pushing forward, stay committed to your goals, and let every fasted workout be a step towards a healthier, more empowered you.

Remember, every journey begins with a single step. Take that step today and start experiencing the transformative power of fasting and exercise. Let your story be one of success, resilience, and profound personal growth.

6
Stress, Anxiety, And Our Inner Calm

I remember the day as if it were yesterday. I was sitting in my office, staring at the computer screen, my heart pounding in my chest. The deadline for a critical project was looming, and I was nowhere near completion. As the minutes ticked by, I could feel the tension rising in my body, my breath becoming shallow and rapid. The stress was overwhelming, consuming my every thought and action.

It's a feeling that many of us know all too well. In the fast-paced, high-pressure world we live in, stress and anxiety have become ubiquitous companions, shadowing our every move. Whether it's the demands of work, the challenges of family life, or the constant pressure to keep up with the ever-changing landscape of our social and cultural norms, stress has become an inescapable part of the modern human experience.

But what exactly is stress, and how does it impact our lives on a fundamental level? At its core, stress is a state of worry or mental tension caused by a difficult situation. It's a natural human response, designed to prompt us to address the challenges and threats that we face in our daily lives. In essence, worry is fear – fear that something might happen, fear that the perception of ourselves might change in the eyes of others or in our own self-image.

So much of the stress we experience can be traced back to these fears about how we are perceived – by our colleagues, our loved ones, and perhaps most importantly, by ourselves. At work, we worry about meeting expectations, maintaining our performance, and achieving success, all the while fearing the specter of failure and the impact it might have on our professional reputation. At home, we feel the weight of our roles and responsibilities, the pressure to be a good parent, spouse, or child, and the fear of not living up to the expectations of those closest to us.

And then there's the ever-present stress of "keeping up

with the Joneses" – the fear of losing our social standing or being perceived as somehow less than our peers. We feel compelled to match or surpass the lifestyle and possessions of those around us, as if these external markers were the ultimate measure of our worth and value as individuals. It's a pressure that can drive us to make choices that may not align with our true needs or desires, all in the name of maintaining a certain image or status.

The toll that this constant stress and anxiety can take on our physical and emotional well-being is profound. When we're stressed, our bodies release cortisol, a hormone that triggers cravings for high-sugar, high-fat foods that provide a momentary sense of comfort and satisfaction, but ultimately leave us feeling worse than before. Stress can wreak havoc on our digestive system, leading to bloating, pain, and indigestion. And over time, chronic stress can contribute to a host of health problems, from heart disease and high blood pressure to depression and anxiety disorders.

But what if there was a way to cultivate the self-discipline and resilience needed to navigate the turbulent waters of stress and anxiety? This is where the practice of intermittent fasting comes in – not as a direct solution to the emotional and psychological roots of stress, but as a powerful tool for developing the inner strength and clarity to confront these challenges head-on.

When I first began my journey with intermittent fasting, I was struck by the profound changes I noticed not just in my physical health, but in my overall sense of well-being. As I learned to listen to my body's natural hunger signals and distinguish between true physical hunger and the emotional cravings that often drove me to eat, I began to feel a sense of control and empowerment that extended far beyond my dietary choices.

The discipline of maintaining a fasting schedule gave me a structure and routine that helped to anchor me in the midst of life's uncertainties. It was a tangible reminder of my own inner strength and resilience, a daily practice that reinforced my ability to overcome challenges and stay true to my goals and values. The act of fasting itself became a powerful metaphor for the kind of mental and emotional discipline that is so essential in navigating the stresses and anxieties of modern life.

Psychological Benefits Of Intermittent Fasting

The process of intermittent fasting is not merely a quest for physical transformation, but a gateway to profound psychological and emotional benefits. Through my exploration of the science behind this ancient practice, it has become clear that our eating patterns are intricately intertwined with our mental well-being. The simple act of fasting can serve as a powerful tool for cultivating resilience, clarity, and inner calm.

At the heart of this connection lies the complex interplay between stress and our eating behaviors. A recent systematic review and meta-analysis published in the journal Health Psychology Review[1] sheds light on this intricate relationship, revealing how stress can profoundly influence our dietary choices and overall health.

The study defines stress as any noxious event or episode in an individual's environment that can be appraised as threatening, risky, or harmful. This definition, rooted in the transactional model of stress, emphasizes the subjective nature of the stress experience, highlighting how it involves an appraisal process where an individual assesses whether an environmental demand exceeds their ability to cope.

When we find ourselves in the grip of stress, a cascade of biological responses is set in motion, chief among

---

[1] Hill, Deborah, Mark Conner, Faye Clancy, Rachael Moss, Sarah Wilding, Matt Bristow, and Daryl B. O'Connor. "Stress and Eating Behaviours in Healthy Adults: A Systematic Review and Meta-Analysis." Health Psychology Review 16, no. 2 (2022): 280-304. https://doi.org/10.1080/17437199.2021.1923406

them the release of the hormone cortisol. Cortisol, often dubbed the "stress hormone," plays a crucial role in regulating our appetite and cravings, particularly for high-fat and high-sugar foods that provide a quick burst of energy and comfort.

It's a response that made perfect sense in the context of our evolutionary past, when stress often signaled a threat to our survival, and the need for readily available energy was paramount. But in the modern world, where stress is more often a product of our mental and emotional landscape than a physical danger, this biological link between stress and unhealthy eating habits can become a maladaptive cycle, perpetuating feelings of anxiety and contributing to poor health outcomes.

This is where the practice of intermittent fasting enters the picture, offering a powerful means of disrupting this cycle and cultivating a greater sense of emotional equilibrium. By consciously choosing to abstain from food for set periods of time, we give ourselves the opportunity to observe and reframe our relationship with stress and the cravings it engenders.

In the quiet space of a fast, free from the constant demands of our appetite, we can begin to cultivate a deeper awareness of the emotional and psychological roots of our hunger. We learn to distinguish between the physical sensations of true hunger and the often-misinterpreted signals of stress, boredom, or anxiety that can drive us to seek solace in food.

This heightened self-awareness is the foundation of the psychological benefits of intermittent fasting. As we become more attuned to our own internal landscape, we develop a greater capacity for self-regulation and emotional resilience. We learn to sit with our discomfort, to observe our cravings without judgment, and to make conscious choices about how we nourish ourselves, both physically and emotionally. Through this practice, we cultivate a sense of mindfulness and presence that extends far beyond our relationship with food, equipping us with the tools to navigate life's inevitable stresses and challenges with greater clarity, purpose, and resilience.

But the benefits of fasting extend beyond the realm of stress management alone. Research has shown that the practice of intermittent fasting can have profound effects on brain health and cognitive function, thanks in part to the production of ketones that occurs when the body is in a fasted state[2].

---

[2] Gudden, Jip, Alejandro Arias Vasquez, and Mirjam Bloemendaal. "The Effects of Intermittent Fasting on Brain and Cognitive Function." Nutrients 13, no. 3166 (2021). https://doi.org/10.3390/nu13093166

These ketones, produced when the body begins to break down stored fat for energy, have been linked to increased levels of BDNF (brain-derived neurotrophic factor), a protein that supports the growth and survival of neurons and enhances neuroplasticity. In essence, the metabolic switch that occurs during fasting may help to create a more adaptable, resilient brain, better equipped to handle the challenges of our fast-paced modern world.

But perhaps the most profound psychological benefit of intermittent fasting lies in the way it can help us to cultivate a greater sense of presence and mindfulness in all aspects of our lives. By learning to observe our hunger with curiosity and non-judgment, we develop a skill that extends far beyond the realm of food and eating.

We begin to approach our thoughts, our emotions, and our experiences with the same sense of openness and acceptance, learning to ride the waves of discomfort and uncertainty with greater ease and grace. In this way, the practice of fasting becomes a powerful tool for personal growth and transformation, a means of cultivating the inner strength and clarity we need to navigate life's challenges with greater equanimity and purpose.

Of course, the pursuit of intermittent fasting is not without its challenges. The pursuit of reframing our relationship with food and hunger can be a daunting one, requiring patience, self-compassion, and a willingness to confront the deep-seated beliefs and patterns that have shaped our eating habits over a lifetime.

But in my experience, the rewards of this endeavour are well worth the effort. As I've learned to embrace the ebb and flow of hunger and satiety, to trust in the wisdom of my body and the resilience of my spirit, I've discovered a sense of freedom and empowerment that extends far beyond the confines of my plate.

The practice of intermittent fasting, when deepened and sustained, naturally cultivates a heightened awareness of our body's physical and emotional signals. This self-awareness is the foundation upon which we can build effective strategies for managing stress and navigating life's challenges with greater resilience and adaptability.

Breathing Exercises

One such strategy that has profoundly impacted my own exploration is the practice of Systema breathing. Like the monster in the 1979 movie Alien, stress can quickly grow from a tiny seed of anxiety into an all-consuming force that takes over our lives. But what if we could spot stress as it is beginning, sprouting like a weed in our carefully tended garden of tranquility? What if we could catch the Alien just as it hatched from the egg, before it had the chance to grow strong and wreak havoc on our well-being?

This is where the power of Systema breathing comes in. Almost by accident, I stumbled upon a little book called "Let Every Breath..." by Vladimir Vasiliev, a manual for this unique approach to breath work. While I have not trained in the Russian martial art of Systema itself, I can passionately recommend its breathing exercises as a tool for recognizing and taming stress in all its forms.

At its core, Systema breathing is based on the understanding that stress is born out of a disruption in our breathing patterns. Breath, it all begins with breath. Stress is born out of a disruption in our breathing! As Vasiliev explains, "You usually disrupt your breathing cycle in response to any stressful factor when something unexpected happens (with your tense mental or physical reaction) or due to psychological habits, such as anxiety and fear. These disruptions may be unconscious reactions to a sudden movement or sound, or an intense emotion. Even simple actions can trigger breath disruptions."[3]

---

[3] Vasiliev, Vladimir. Let Every Breath: Secrets of the Russian Breath Masters. Toronto, Canada: Russian Martial Art, 2006

By learning to identify and correct these disruptions through simple yet powerful breathing exercises, we can effectively regulate our body's stress response and cultivate a greater sense of calm and emotional balance. And as we'll explore in the coming pages, this heightened awareness of our breath and its connection to our mental and emotional states is a natural complement to the practice of intermittent fasting, enhancing the transformative potential of both disciplines.

What I appreciate about the exercises presented in this book is their simplicity and accessibility. The postures and exercises are straightforward, requiring no complicated positions. The purpose is to better understand your body. Systema breathing simulates daily stresses in life and allows you to overcome and manage them through breathing. The object is to breathe right, relaxed. Relaxation implies absence of fear. Absence of fear is absence of stress.

One particularly powerful exercise is designed to be performed the moment you wake up, still lying in bed. It's a great way to start your day:

1. Position: Start by lying in bed on your back, with your arms at your sides and legs naturally extended. Ensure your head and neck are comfortably positioned.
2. Inhale and Tense: Begin by slowly inhaling through

your nose. As you do so, gradually tense every muscle in your body, starting from your toes and moving up to your head. Squeeze the muscles tightly but not to the point of discomfort.

3. Hold and Intensify: Hold your breath for a moment with your body fully tensed. Intensify the tension slightly if possible, ensuring it is still comfortable.

4. Exhale and Relax: Slowly exhale through your mouth and simultaneously release the tension in your muscles, starting from your head and moving down to your toes. Feel the relaxation spreading as you exhale.

5. Repeat: You can repeat this cycle a few times. With each repetition, focus on the feeling of tension as you inhale and the sense of relaxation as you exhale.

This exercise helps wake up the body, increases your awareness of muscle states, and enhances control over tension and relaxation. It's a simple yet effective way to activate your muscles and prepare your body and mind for the day ahead.

Another powerful exercise is the "breathing pyramid," designed to integrate controlled breathing with walking:

1. Start Walking: Begin walking at a comfortable, steady pace. The goal is to synchronize your steps with your breathing in a gradually increasing and then decreasing

pattern.

2. Initial Breathing Steps: Start by inhaling through your nose for one step, then exhale through your mouth for one step. This is the base of the pyramid.

3. Increase the Count: On the next cycle, inhale for two steps and then exhale for two steps. Continue increasing the count of your steps during inhalation and exhalation until you reach a maximum number that feels comfortable. Typically, this might go up to five or six steps per breath, depending on your lung capacity and walking speed.

4. Reverse the Pattern: After reaching your maximum comfortable breath count, start decreasing the count. If you went up to five steps per breath, go down to four steps per breath in the next cycle, then three, and so forth, until you are back to one step per breath.

5. Focus on Smooth Transition: Ensure that the transitions between inhaling and exhaling are smooth. Try not to hold your breath at any point; maintain a steady, continuous flow of breathing.

6. Repeat the Pyramid: You can repeat the pyramid pattern as many times as you like during your walk. This exercise helps in developing lung capacity, control over your breathing, and a rhythmic synchronization between your breath and steps.

For me, the biggest discovery in performing this exercise occurred when I reached steps 3 or 4 of the pyramid. The physical sensations in my body strongly resembled those I experience when I'm stressed or irritable. The key lesson here is to acknowledge these physical sensations during moments of stress and understand that you can overcome them through the simple act of mindful breathing.

Recognizing how the physical sensations experienced during a structured exercise like the "breathing pyramid" mirror those you encounter during stress or irritation is crucial. It highlights an important aspect of stress management—awareness of your body's responses.

When you're aware of how your body physically manifests stress, you can use controlled breathing as a practical tool to mitigate these responses. Breathing exercises help regulate the body's stress response by activating the parasympathetic nervous system, which slows the heart rate and lowers blood pressure, thereby promoting a state of calmness.

The lesson from this experience with the exercise suggests a powerful strategy: by consciously altering your breathing pattern, you can directly influence your emotional and physical state. This is a technique that can be applied in real-world situations where stress or irritability arises. Instead of being overwhelmed by these feelings, you can engage in mindful breathing to regain control and achieve a more relaxed state. This approach not only helps in managing the immediate stress response but also enhances overall emotional resilience.

This heightened awareness and ability to regulate stress through breathing has been a natural complement to my process with intermittent fasting. As I've become more attuned to my body's signals through the practice of fasting, I've also developed a keener sense of the subtle cues that indicate the onset of stress or emotional hunger.

I recall one particular instance where this awareness was put to the test. It was late in the afternoon, and I was in the midst of a challenging work project. I could feel the familiar tension creeping into my shoulders and temples, my breath becoming shallow and constricted. In the past, I might have reached for a snack or lashed out at someone as a way to cope with the mounting stress, mistaking my emotional discomfort for physical hunger.

But armed with the tools of mindful breathing and the heightened body awareness cultivated through fasting, I chose a different path. Instead of reacting impulsively to the urge to eat or lash out, I took a moment to pause and observe the sensations arising in my body. I noticed the tightness in my chest, the racing of my thoughts, and the subtle gnawing sensation in my stomach that I might have previously interpreted as hunger.

Recognizing these stress signals, I stepped away from my desk and took a five-minute walk around the office, practicing my breath pyramid. With each step, I focused on synchronizing my breath with my movements, gradually increasing and then decreasing the number of steps per breath. As I progressed through the exercise, I could feel the tension begin to dissipate, my mind growing clearer and more focused.

By the time I returned to my desk, the stress signals in my body had significantly diminished. I recognized that what I had been feeling was not true physical hunger, but rather a conditioned response to stress. By simply observing these sensations without judgment and engaging in a mindful breathing exercise, I was able to ride out the wave of discomfort, knowing that it would eventually pass.

This experience was a powerful reminder of the ways in which fasting and mindful breathing can work synergistically to enhance our overall well-being. By cultivating a deeper awareness of our physical and emotional states, we can learn to respond to life's challenges with greater equanimity and resilience.

Mindful eating, then, becomes an extension of this

practice – a way of bringing the same level of attention and presence to our relationship with food. When we eat mindfully, we're not just nourishing our bodies, but also nurturing a deeper connection with ourselves and the world around us.

We learn to savor each bite, to appreciate the flavors, textures, and aromas of our food, and to listen closely to the subtle cues of hunger and satiety. We become more attuned to the ways in which our emotional states can influence our eating habits, and we develop the skills to navigate these challenges with greater ease and self-compassion.

In this way, the practice of intermittent fasting becomes a gateway to a more mindful, embodied way of living. By learning to listen deeply to the wisdom of our bodies and to trust in the innate intelligence of our hunger and fullness cues, we open ourselves up to a richer, more nourishing experience of life itself.

Exploring the practice of intermittent fasting, I've come to understand that the challenges we face along the way are not merely obstacles to be overcome, but opportunities for profound personal growth and transformation. Each moment of discomfort, each craving resisted, becomes a chance to cultivate greater resilience and self-awareness, to build the mental and emotional muscles that will serve us well in all areas of our lives.

I remember the early days of my fasting exploration, when the hunger pangs would come in waves, threatening to derail my resolve. There were times when I would find myself standing in front of the fridge, hand poised on the handle, fighting an internal battle between my desire for food and my commitment to my fasting protocol.

In those moments, it would have been easy to give in, to tell myself that one small snack wouldn't make a difference. But I knew that the real challenge wasn't the physical sensation of hunger, but the mental and emotional discomfort that came with it. By learning to sit with that discomfort, to observe it with curiosity and compassion, I was slowly building the resilience and self-trust that would become the foundation of my fasting practice.

Over time, as I continued to navigate the ups and downs of my fasting adventure, I began to notice a profound shift in my overall relationship with anxiety and stress. The challenges I faced in my fasting practice – the moments of hunger, the social pressures, the doubts and fears – became a microcosm of the larger challenges I faced in my life.

Just as I had learned to meet my hunger with mindfulness and equanimity, I found myself better equipped to navigate the inevitable stresses and uncertainties of daily life. When anxiety would arise, I could meet it with the same curiosity and non-judgment that I brought to my fasting practice, knowing that it, too, would eventually pass.

This is not to say that the quest of intermittent fasting is always easy or comfortable. As with any new habit or lifestyle change, there are bound to be moments of doubt, fear, and resistance. Many people, when first starting out with fasting, find themselves grappling with a host of common anxieties and concerns.

There may be a fear of hunger, a worry that the physical sensations of an empty stomach will be too much to bear. There may be concerns about social eating, a fear of missing out on meals with friends and loved ones or of being judged for one's food choices. And there may be doubts about one's own ability to stick with the practice, to navigate the inevitable challenges and setbacks that arise along the way.

To these fears and anxieties, I offer the same advice that has served me well on my own fasting endeavor: approach the practice with curiosity, compassion, and a willingness to learn. Know that the discomfort you feel is not a sign of failure, but an opportunity for growth and self-discovery.

When hunger arises, meet it with mindfulness and breath, knowing that it is a temporary sensation that will eventually pass. When social pressures or temptations arise, remember the deeper reasons why you chose to embark on this pursuit – the desire for greater health, vitality, and self-awareness.

And when doubts or setbacks arise, as they inevitably will, meet them with self-compassion and a renewed commitment to your practice. Remember that the endeavor of intermittent fasting is not about perfection, but about progress – about showing up each day with an open heart and a willingness to learn.

Reflecting on my endeavor with intermittent fasting, I am struck by the profound ways in which this simple practice has transformed not just my physical health, but my entire relationship with myself and the world around me. What began as a way to lose weight and improve my body composition has become a gateway to a deeper sense of mental clarity, emotional resilience, and spiritual well-being.

Through the challenges and triumphs of my fasting practice, I have learned to trust in the wisdom of my body, to listen to its subtle cues and signals with greater attunement and respect. I have discovered a new sense of empowerment and self-control, a feeling that I am capable of making choices that align with my deepest values and aspirations.

So to those who may be considering embarking on their own fasting journey, I invite you to approach the practice with an open heart and a curious mind. Know that the path may not always be easy, but that the rewards – the increased vitality, the mental clarity, the emotional resilience – are well worth the effort.

As you navigate the inevitable ups and downs of your own fasting practice, remember to be kind to yourself, to celebrate your successes and learn from your setbacks. And above all, trust in the wisdom of your own body and the power of your own spirit to guide you towards a deeper sense of health, happiness, and wholeness.

In a world that can often feel overwhelming and stressful, the practice of intermittent fasting offers a powerful tool for reclaiming our physical, mental, and emotional well-being. By learning to harmonize our eating patterns with the natural rhythms of our bodies and minds, we open ourselves up to a greater sense of balance, resilience, and inner peace. So let us embrace this transformative adventure with courage, compassion, and a deep commitment to our own self-care, trusting in the ancient wisdom of fasting to guide us towards a brighter, more vibrant future. And let us remember that, no matter where we are on our own process to wellness, we are never alone – we are part of a larger community of seekers, all striving towards greater health, happiness, and wholeness.

7
Fasting, Sleep, And Food Choices

My fasting journey has been a revelatory experience, unlocking not just the physical benefits of improved health and vitality, but a profound transformation in my relationship with myself, my body, and the world around me. As I've navigated the ebb and flow of hunger and satiety, I've come to appreciate the complex ways in which our eating patterns are interwoven with the very fabric of our lives – our sleep, our emotional well-being, and the choices we make in nourishing ourselves.

In the previous chapters, we've explored the evolutionary wisdom inherent in the ancient rhythms of feast and famine, and how embracing these cycles can unlock a wellspring of resilience and self-awareness. Going deeper into the practice of intermittent fasting, I've come to realize that the true power of this endeavor lies not just in the physical changes it catalyzes, but in the profound impact it can have on our overall quality of life.

It all began with those first tentative steps, compressing my eating window by simply delaying my breakfast and moving my dinner a bit earlier. By doing so, I managed to get 12 hours of fasting in each day. Weekends were off, as I had no fasting routine during those times. At first, I'll admit, there was a nagging sense of worry – a fear that somehow, this deprivation of food would be harmful, that my body would rebel against the change. But as the days turned into weeks, I was surprised to find that my body adapted with remarkable ease, the initial discomfort giving way to a newfound sense of energy and clarity.

The real turning point came when I made the decision to cut dinner altogether, opting instead for a hearty breakfast and a substantial lunch. This was a profound shift, not just in my eating habits, but in my very relationship with food. For years, I had fallen into the routine of dinner as a matter of course, without ever truly considering whether I was hungry or not. It was dinner time, so I ate – end of story. But now, with the freedom of a compressed feeding window, I found myself attuned to the subtle cues of my body, no longer mindlessly consuming out of habit or obligation.

The changes I experienced were palpable, and they extended far beyond the physical realm. I noticed that my snoring had diminished as well, a testament to the profound impact that our eating habits can have on our overall sleep quality and respiratory function. It was as if my body, no longer burdened by the constant demands of digestion, was finally able to settle into a state of deep, rejuvenating rest.

This journey has been a profound exploration of the interconnectedness of the various facets of our health and well-being. The choices we make in nourishing ourselves, the rhythms we establish in our sleep patterns, and the ways in which we navigate the ebb and flow of hunger and satiety – all of these elements are inextricably linked, weaving a tapestry of wellness that is unique to each individual.

As we continue to explore the transformative power of intermittent fasting, I invite you to join me in a deeper exploration of this intricate web of relationships. Together, let us uncover the secrets that lie beneath the surface of our sleep, our food choices, and the subtle cues of our bodies – for in doing so, we just might unlock the keys to a more vibrant, balanced, and joyful way of living.

Fasting and Sleep Quality

The research on the relationship between intermittent fasting and sleep quality provides compelling insights into the profound ways in which these two elements of our health and well-being are interconnected. As the study "Eat, Train, Sleep—Retreat? Hormonal Interactions of Intermittent Fasting, Exercise and Circadian Rhythm"[1] explains, intermittent fasting can have a profound impact on our circadian rhythms – the internal biological clocks that govern our sleep-wake cycles and other physiological processes. By restricting our eating to a specific window of time, we help reinforce the alignment of these natural rhythms with the environmental cues of light and dark. This synchronization is crucial for maintaining a consistent, high-quality sleep pattern, as it allows our bodies to anticipate and respond to these natural cycles, facilitating the release of key hormones like melatonin, which promotes sleep, and cortisol, which helps regulate our wakefulness.

---

[1] Haupt, Sandra, Max L. Eckstein, Alina Wolf, Rebecca T. Zimmer, Nadine B. Wachsmuth, and Othmar Moser. 2021. "Eat, Train, Sleep—Retreat? Hormonal Interactions of Intermittent Fasting, Exercise and Circadian Rhythm." Biomolecules 11, no. 4 (April): 516. https://doi.org/10.3390/biom11040516

The study also sheds light on the two-way street between our body's main clock and the smaller clocks found in various organs and tissues. When the main clock in our brain falls out of sync or when the metabolic processes in our body are thrown off balance, it can lead to disruptions in our natural daily rhythms. This is where intermittent fasting comes in – by helping to realign these internal clocks with the external world around us, fasting creates a sense of harmony between the different systems that keep us healthy and thriving.

In simpler terms, our body has a master clock that keeps everything running smoothly, but it also relies on smaller clocks throughout our organs to stay in tune. These smaller clocks, known as peripheral clocks, can be found in places like the liver and pancreas. The liver clock, for example, helps regulate the production of glucose and the breakdown of fats, while the pancreas clock plays a role in controlling the release of insulin. If any of these clocks are out of whack, it can throw off our entire system, leading to metabolic imbalances and even chronic diseases. Intermittent fasting acts as a reset button, helping to synchronize all of these clocks and keep them working together in perfect harmony. By aligning our eating patterns with the natural rhythms of day and night, we're essentially giving our body the cues it needs to function at its best, promoting better health and well-being from the inside out.

Just as we rely on the rising and setting of the sun to guide our daily activities, our body's clocks rely on the timing of our meals to stay in sync. By embracing the practice of intermittent fasting, we're tapping into this ancient wisdom and allowing our bodies to find their natural rhythm once again.

The study "Fasting, Circadian Rhythms, and Time-Restricted Feeding in Healthy Lifespan"[2] introduces another fascinating approach to aligning our eating patterns with our circadian rhythms: time-restricted feeding (TRF). TRF involves consuming all daily calories within a specific window of time, usually 12 hours or less, without explicitly altering the quantity or quality of the diet. This practice has shown promise in both animal and human studies, with potential benefits ranging from weight loss and improved sleep quality to reduced inflammation and enhanced metabolic health. The study also highlights the prevalence and consequences of circadian disruption in modern society. Our 24/7 lifestyles, characterized by artificial light exposure, erratic eating patterns, and chronic stress, can wreak havoc on our internal clocks, leading to a host of health issues, including obesity, metabolic syndrome, and even cancer. By embracing practices like intermittent fast-

---

2 Longo, Valter D., and Satchidananda Panda. 2016. "Fasting, Circadian Rhythms, and Time-Restricted Feeding in Healthy Lifespan." Cell Metabolism 23, no. 6 (June 14): 1048-1059. https://doi.org/10.1016/j.cmet.2016.06.001

ing and TRF, we have the power to reset these disrupted rhythms and restore a sense of balance to our bodies and minds.

It's important to note, however, that the optimal approach to fasting may vary depending on an individual's age, life stage, and unique health status. As the study points out, the effects of dietary interventions like fasting can differ between young and old organisms, underscoring the need for personalized, age-specific recommendations. Moreover, each individual should experiment by slowly beginning to compress their feeding window to find a time interval for ingesting food that best suits their lifestyle, preferences, and body's response. This process of self-discovery is crucial, as there is no one-size-fits-all approach to intermittent fasting. It's also essential for anyone with special health conditions or concerns to consult with their physician before embarking on any fasting regimen, to ensure that the chosen approach is safe and appropriate for their specific needs.

As I've personally experienced, the impact of fasting on my sleep has been nothing short of transformative. Gone are the days of tossing and turning, plagued by the discomfort of acid reflux and the persistent hum of my own snoring. Instead, I find myself drifting off to sleep with ease, my body and mind in a state of harmonious alignment, ready to reap the benefits of deep, rejuvenating slumber.

It's a testament to the power of this ancient practice, and the ways in which it can unlock a new level of vitality and well-being in our lives. By tuning in to the natural rhythms of our bodies and honoring the ebb and flow of our hunger and satiety, we open ourselves up to a world of possibilities – a world where our sleep, our energy, and our overall sense of balance are all elevated to new heights.

Food Cravings and Choices

Exploring the transformative power of intermittent fasting reveals its profound impact on our relationship with food. Through my own journey, I've discovered that fasting is not just a means of optimizing our physical health, but also a powerful tool for cultivating self-awareness and making choices that align with our deepest values and aspirations.

My love affair with food began at a young age, instilled in me by my mother, a master in the kitchen. Her generosity and passion for cooking had a profound impact on me, and I came to associate the act of eating with expressions of love, comfort, and gratitude. As a child, I learned that to truly show appreciation for a dish, one had to eat to the point of bursting, that fullness was a sign of love and respect for the person who prepared the meal. This unconscious pattern of behavior followed me into adulthood, shaping my relationship with food for many years.

It wasn't until I embarked on the path of intermittent fasting that I began to unravel these deeply ingrained habits and beliefs, to question the assumptions that had long governed my approach to nourishment. At first, the freedom of the fasting window felt like a revelation – a chance to eat to my heart's content, without the constraints of portion control or calorie counting. It was a relief to know that I could indulge in the foods I loved, that I could honor my mother's legacy of generosity and abundance at the table.

However, as I progressed in my practice of intermittent fasting, I began to notice a subtle shift in my relationship with food. I found myself tuning in to the subtle signals of my body, learning to distinguish between true hunger and the emotional or habitual drivers that had long governed my eating patterns. Through this process, I recognized the unconscious beliefs and behaviors around food that I had carried with me since childhood. Slowly, I began to establish healthier boundaries around my eating, learning to honor my hunger without crossing the line into discomfort or overindulgence. I learned to serve myself smaller portions, to savor each bite with mindfulness and presence, and to trust that my body would tell me when it had enough.

Progressing further, I cultivated a deeper awareness of my own needs and desires, which led to a profound shift in my food cravings and preferences.. Foods that had once held an irresistible allure – the greasy burgers and fast-food indulgences of my past – no longer called to me with the same intensity. Instead, I found myself drawn to the vibrant flavors and textures of whole, nourishing foods – the crisp snap of a fresh vegetable, the succulent juiciness of a perfectly grilled piece of meat. It was as if my body, freed from the constant onslaught of processed and artificial ingredients, was finally able to speak its truth – to guide me towards the foods that would truly nourish and sustain me. And as I learned to listen to these cues with greater attunement and respect, I discovered a newfound sense of balance and harmony in my relationship with food.

As you progress in your fasting window, it's important to ask yourself: How satisfied am I with what I ate? How full am I? Notice any instances of bloating, acidity, gas, burping, etc. Which food caused these symptoms? Was it a single food or a combination? When was my hunger peak time, at what time was I the hungriest? Was my hunger a true need for nourishment or a craving? If you identify your hunger peak time not related to anxiety, is it worth trying to modify your feeding window to include this hunger peak time? This does not mean fasting for fewer hours, but simply adjusting your feeding window to your own natural rhythms.

In my own journey, when I first made the decision to skip dinner, my feeding window included breakfast and lunch. However, by listening to my body's signals and peak hunger times, I started to shift my feeding window. Nowadays, I don't ingest any food before noon, as I've found that this approach aligns better with my body's natural rhythms and leads to greater overall satisfaction and well-being.

This experience of tuning into my body's needs and adjusting my fasting window accordingly was just one of the many profound insights I gained through my fasting journey. Perhaps the most profound revelation came in the way that fasting allowed me to fully appreciate the impact of different foods on my body and mind. By giving my digestive system the time and space to process each meal completely before introducing another, I was able to observe with startling clarity the ways in which certain foods or combinations of ingredients affected my physical and emotional well-being.

I noticed how certain foods left me feeling bloated and uncomfortable, while others filled me with a sense of lightness and vitality. As a quick example, I discovered that the thirst I experienced after consuming garlic and red wine together was a unique reaction to that specific combination, and not something that occurred when I consumed them separately.

Through this process of experimentation and self-observation, I came to understand that the key to true nourishment lies not in any one-size-fits-all approach, but in the cultivation of a deep and abiding self-awareness. By learning to listen to the language of our own bodies, to honor the unique needs and preferences that make us who we are, we open ourselves up to a world of possibilities – a world where food becomes not just a source of sustenance, but a pathway to greater self-understanding and self-love.

As we continue to explore the transformative power of intermittent fasting, I invite you to join me in this process of self-discovery. Approach your relationship with food with curiosity and compassion, listen to the subtle cues and signals that your body sends you, and trust in the innate wisdom that lies within. For in doing so, we open ourselves up to a world of possibilities – a world where nourishment becomes not just a matter of what we put into our bodies, but a reflection of the love and care we show ourselves. A world where our food choices become a powerful tool for self-discovery and self-transformation, guiding us towards a life of greater vitality, balance, and joy.

Reflecting on my own fasting journey, I am struck by the profound ways in which this practice has transformed my relationship with food and my body. Beyond the physical benefits of improved sleep quality and increased energy levels, fasting has also brought about significant mental and emotional shifts. Through the daily practice of delaying gratification and tuning into my body's needs, I have cultivated a deeper sense of self-discipline, resilience, and adaptability. These qualities have spilled over into other areas of my life, empowering me to face challenges with greater ease and confidence.

I invite you to view fasting not as a restrictive diet or a set of rigid rules, but as a powerful tool for reclaiming your health and well-being. By embracing the discomfort of hunger and learning to distinguish between true nourishment and fleeting cravings, you are taking a stand for your own self-care and self-respect. You are sending a message to yourself and to the world that you are worthy of vibrant health, boundless energy, and a joyful relationship with food.

As we come to the end of this chapter, I hope that the insights and experiences I have shared have inspired you to approach your own fasting journey with curiosity, compassion, and an open mind. Remember that the path to optimal health and well-being is unique to each individual, and that fasting is just one tool in your self-care toolkit. What works for me may not work for you, and that's okay. The most important thing is to stay attuned to your own body's needs and to approach each day with a willingness to learn and grow.

Throughout this chapter, we have explored the interconnectedness of fasting, sleep, and food choices, and how each of these elements plays a crucial role in our overall health and happiness. By prioritizing restful sleep, nourishing our bodies with whole, unprocessed foods, and allowing ourselves the space to experience true hunger and satiety, we are laying the foundation for a lifetime of vibrant health and well-being.

So as you embark on your own fasting journey, remember to be patient with yourself, to celebrate your successes, and to view each challenge as an opportunity for growth and self-discovery. Trust in the wisdom of your own body, and know that you have the power within you to create the health and happiness you deserve.

8
Finding Your Middle Way

Embarking on the final chapter of our transformative journey into the world of intermittent fasting, we must acknowledge a profound truth that underlies this ancient practice: the path of fasting is not a one-size-fits-all prescription, but a deeply personal pilgrimage of self-discovery and transformation. Just as each of us bears the unique imprint of our individual histories, goals, and circumstances, so too must our approach to fasting be tailored to the singular landscape of our own lives.

In the pages that follow, we will explore the art and science of crafting a fasting practice that is uniquely your own, one that honors your distinct needs, aspirations, and challenges. As you forge your own path through the wilderness of fasting, you may just discover that the destination is less important than the journey itself. For in the end, the goal is not simply to achieve a particular number on the scale or a specific set of health metrics, but to unlock a deeper sense of vitality, resilience, and wholeness that permeates every aspect of your being.

So let us set forth on this final leg of our expedition with open hearts and curious minds, ready to embrace the discomfort and the discovery, the triumphs and the setbacks, knowing that each step brings us closer to the fullest expression of our potential. For in the end, the fasting progression is not just about changing our bodies, but about transforming our lives – a profound and sacred journey that leads us back to the deepest truth of who we are and forward to a vision of the vibrant, thriving beings we were always meant to be.

Beginning on Your Fasting Journey

As we stand on the threshold of this fasting journey, I am reminded of the old adage that every voyage begins with a single step. And yet, the path that stretches before each of us is as unique as the footprints we will leave behind.

In my own way, I have come to understand that fasting is not merely a protocol to be followed, but a deeply personal exploration of the mind, body, and spirit. It is a path that demands we show up fully, with all of our fears and doubts, our hopes and aspirations, our unique strengths and vulnerabilities.

As you take your first steps on this path, remember that there will be moments of discomfort and uncertainty, times when the old habits and patterns that have long governed your relationship with food will rise up to challenge your resolve. In these moments, remember that growth often lies on the other side of resistance, that the temporary discomfort of change is the price we pay for the profound rewards of transformation.

Embrace the fact that what works for one person may not work for another, and that is okay. The beauty of this path is that it invites us to tune into the subtle language of our own bodies and minds, to develop a deep and abiding trust in the wisdom that lies within. Beneath the surface of our individual goals and aspirations, there lies a common yearning for transformation.

For some, this may manifest as a deep desire to shed the physical and emotional burdens that have accumulated over years of unhealthy habits and patterns. For others, the fasting process may be a quest for greater mental clarity and focus, a way to pierce through the veil of distraction and noise that so often clouds our perception in this modern age. And for still others, fasting may represent a spiritual pilgrimage, an opportunity to cultivate a deeper sense of connection and alignment with the rhythms of the natural world.

So as you commence on this course, let go of any assumed notions or rigid expectations. Allow yourself the freedom to experiment, to make mistakes, to learn and grow and adapt as you go. Approach each day with a beginner's mind, free from the weight of expectation or comparison. Let go of any preconceived notions of what fasting "should" look like, and remember that the true magic of fasting lies not in the destination, but in the road itself. It is in the daily practice of showing up, of honoring your own unique needs and rhythms, of learning to trust in the innate intelligence of your own being.

As you contemplate embarking on your fasting journey, it is essential to take a moment to reflect on the deeper purpose that propels you forward. To harness this potential, however, requires a clear and compelling vision of what you hope to achieve. It is not enough to simply go through the motions, to follow the prescribed protocols and hope for the best. Rather, you must dive deep into the heart of your own desires, to uncover the authentic yearnings that will fuel your endeavor and imbue it with meaning.

So I invite you now to take a pause, to turn inward and contemplate the seeds of intention that you wish to plant in the fertile soil of your fasting practice. Let yourself be guided by questions such as:

What do you hope to gain from fasting, beyond the mere physical benefits of improved health and vitality? Is it a greater sense of emotional well-being, a more harmonious relationship with your own body and mind? Is it a deeper connection to your spiritual path, a way to cultivate the clarity and presence that will allow you to more fully align with your highest purpose?

What aspects of your current lifestyle do you wish to transform through the alchemy of fasting? Are there habits or patterns that no longer serve you, that keep you feeling stuck or stagnant? Are there ways in which you have been living out of alignment with your deepest values and truths, and if so, how might fasting help you to shed the old and embrace the new?

And perhaps most importantly, how can the practice of fasting support your overall vision for a balanced, fulfilling life? What does that life look like, in its most radiant and expansive form? And how might the challenges and triumphs of your fasting pursuit serve as a microcosm for the greater journey of your own becoming?

As you contemplate these questions, I encourage you to take pen to paper and give voice to the stirrings of your soul. For there is something powerful about the act of writing down our goals and aspirations, of giving them concrete form and substance. It is a way of signaling to the universe that we are ready to take the leap, to commit ourselves fully to the path of progression.

And yet, even as you give shape to your intentions, remember to hold them lightly, with a sense of openness and curiosity. For the fasting course is not a linear path, but a winding road full of unexpected detours and revelations. What you set out to achieve may shift and evolve as you go, as you peel back the layers of your own being and discover new depths of understanding and possibility.

So let your goals and motivations be a starting point, a compass to guide you forward, but not a rigid destination that limits your horizons. Trust that, as you surrender to the wisdom of your own body and soul, as you show up each day with a spirit of presence and willingness, the unfolding of your quest will be more beautiful and profound than anything you could have imagined.

Ultimately, the true goal of fasting extends beyond achieving external metrics of success. It is a journey of self-discovery, a path that leads you back to your authentic self, stripped of the layers of conditioning and fear that may have obscured your inner truth. Through this process, you can step forth into the world as a more empowered, resilient, and radiant version of yourself.

As you embark on your fasting journey, one of the first decisions you'll face is choosing the approach that aligns best with your unique goals, lifestyle, and temperament. There are many effective ways to harness the transformative power of fasting, and the key is to find the method that resonates most deeply with you.

Some of the most popular methods include the 12-hour fast, where you restrict your eating window to a 12-hour period each day; the 16:8 approach, which involves fasting for 16 hours and eating within an 8-hour window; the 5:2 method, where you eat normally for five days and significantly reduce your calorie intake on the other two days; and the OMAD, or "one meal a day" approach, where you compress your eating into a single, satisfying meal each day.

In my own path, I began with a simple 12-hour fast, gradually extending my fasting window until I found myself naturally gravitating towards the OMAD approach. There was something profoundly liberating about the simplicity and clarity of this method, the way it allowed me to fully immerse myself in the experience of fasting without the constant distraction of meal planning and preparation.

And yet, as I continued to experiment and refine my practice, I discovered that a combination of OMAD and 18:6 fasting felt most sustainable and nourishing for my own unique needs and rhythms. By alternating between these two approaches, I was able to strike a balance between the intensity of a full-day fast and the gentler rhythm of a shorter eating window, allowing my body and mind to find their own natural equilibrium.

But the truth is, there is no one-size-fits-all approach to fasting, no single method that will work for everyone. What feels nourishing and sustainable for one person may feel restrictive and depleting for another, and the only way to discover your own optimal approach is through a process of gentle experimentation and self-examination.

So as you contemplate the various fasting methods available to you, ask yourself: What feels most aligned with your natural rhythms and preferences? What approach sparks a sense of eagerness and excitement, rather than dread or deprivation? Remember, the true magic of fasting lies not in the specific protocol you follow, but in the way you show up for the process itself. It lies in your willingness to be present with the discomfort and the discovery, to embrace the ebb and flow of hunger and satiety, and to trust in the unfolding of your own unique path.

Overcoming Challenges and Obstacles

It's important to acknowledge that challenges and obstacles are a natural and inevitable part of the fasting process. Whether it's the physical discomfort of hunger, the social pressure to eat in certain situations, or the internal voice of self-doubt and resistance, these challenges can feel overwhelming at times, threatening to derail your progress and undermine your commitment to the practice.

But what if we were to view these obstacles not as roadblocks to be avoided, but as opportunities for growth and self-discovery? What if each moment of discomfort or resistance was an invitation to deepen our understanding of ourselves and our relationship with food, to cultivate greater resilience and self-awareness in the face of life's challenges?

In my own fasting journey, I've encountered my fair share of obstacles and setbacks. There have been times when hunger felt all-consuming, when the thought of going without food for even a few more hours seemed impossible. In these moments, it's essential to remember that these intense sensations are temporary and that our bodies are capable of adapting to short periods of fasting. By staying mindful of our physical and emotional states, and by practicing self-compassion, we can learn to ride out these waves of discomfort and maintain our commitment to our fasting goals.

Another common challenge that many of us face is navigating social situations while fasting. Whether it's attending a dinner party or celebrating a special occasion with friends and family, the pressure to eat and conform to social norms can be intense. However, I've found that a little bit of planning and flexibility can go a long way in helping me stay true to my fasting practice without feeling like an outsider or drawing unnecessary attention to myself.

One strategy that has worked well for me is to simply adjust my fasting hours to accommodate social events and gatherings. If I know I'll be attending a party or dinner with friends, I'll plan ahead and shift my eating window so that it aligns with the time I'll be socializing. This way, I can enjoy the company of others and participate in the festivities without feeling deprived or self-conscious about my fasting practice.

I've also found that there's no need to go out of my way to announce or explain my fasting to others in these situations. By acting normally and engaging in conversation and activities as I would in any other setting, I'm able to stay true to my own goals and values without drawing undue attention or making others feel uncomfortable.

At the end of the day, I've learned that the key to overcoming obstacles and navigating social situations while fasting is to approach them with flexibility, self-awareness, and a commitment to my own goals and values. By finding creative solutions and staying true to myself, I'm able to stay on track with my fasting practice while still enjoying the richness and connection of social experiences.

As you navigate the challenges of your own fasting journey, remember that within you lies a wellspring of strength and wisdom that is greater than any obstacle you may face. By learning to trust in that inner guidance, to meet each challenge with interest and compassion, you open yourself up to a world of possibility and transformation that extends far beyond the realm of fasting alone.

Let us embrace the challenges and obstacles of this journey, not as barriers to be overcome, but as invitations to grow and evolve in ways we never could have imagined. Let us approach each moment of discomfort or resistance as an opportunity to deepen our self-awareness, to cultivate greater resilience, and to trust in the inherent wisdom of our own bodies and minds.

In doing so, we not only strengthen our commitment to our fasting practice but also develop the skills and mindset necessary to navigate life's challenges with greater ease and grace. We learn to approach obstacles with curiosity and compassion, to find creative solutions that align with our values and goals, and to trust in the transformative power of our own inner strength and wisdom.

So as you continue on your fasting journey, remember that the challenges you face are not simply hurdles to be overcome, but precious opportunities for growth, self-discovery, and transformation. Embrace them with an open heart and a curious mind, and trust that each step, each setback, each triumph, is an essential part of your unique path toward greater health, happiness, and wholeness.

Beyond Fasting - A Life in Balance

As we've explored throughout this chapter, the practice of fasting is a powerful tool in a holistic approach to well-being, creating a ripple effect of balance and vitality that extends far beyond the physical realm. However, to truly harness the transformative potential of fasting, it's essential to approach the practice with a mindset of mindfulness and self-compassion.

Two key concepts that can guide us on this journey are non-attachment and the middle way. Non-attachment encourages us to let go of our fixation on specific outcomes and instead embrace the present moment with openness and curiosity. When applied to the fasting journey, this principle can help us release rigid expectations and approach the practice with a spirit of exploration and self-discovery.

Similarly, the idea of the middle way emphasizes the importance of finding balance and moderation in all aspects of life. By letting go of extreme or restrictive approaches in favor of a more sustainable, nuanced practice, we honor our individual needs and circumstances while still reaping the profound benefits of fasting.

Alongside these guiding principles, the practical techniques of Systema breathing can offer valuable support. The breathing exercises mimic the daily stresses we encounter and help us manage them through controlled breathing. The goal is to breathe in a relaxed and correct manner. Being relaxed means being free from fear, and without fear, there is no stress.

This increased awareness and capacity to manage stress through breathing has naturally enhanced my intermittent fasting journey. As I've grown more sensitive to my body's signals while fasting, I've also sharpened my ability to detect subtle signs of stress or emotional hunger.

Ultimately, by integrating the principles of non-attachment, the middle way, and the practical tools of Systema breathing into our fasting journey, we open ourselves up to a transformative path of self-discovery and personal growth. We learn to trust in the wisdom of our own bodies and minds, to cultivate a deeper sense of resilience and adaptability, and to approach each moment with a sense of curiosity, compassion, and open-hearted presence.

As you embark on your own fasting journey, remember that there is no one "right" way to fast and that the path to optimal well-being is a deeply individual one, shaped by your unique needs, goals, and experiences. Embrace the challenges and setbacks as opportunities for learning and growth, and trust in the wisdom of your own body and mind to guide you towards the practices and rhythms that best serve your highest good.

For in the end, the transformative power of fasting lies not just in the physical benefits it bestows, but in the way it challenges us to confront our deepest beliefs and patterns around food, our bodies, and our lives. It is a practice that invites us to let go of that which no longer serves us, to cultivate a deeper sense of presence and purpose, and to step boldly into the unknown, trusting in the boundless potential that lies within.

So let us embrace this journey with open hearts and curious minds, knowing that each step we take, each challenge we face, each moment of insight and growth, is a sacred part of the unfolding of our highest selves. May your fasting journey be a source of nourishment, inspiration, and transformation, and may it lead you ever closer to the life of balance, purpose, and joy that you so richly deserve.

As you embark on this transformative journey of fasting, remember that every challenge you face, every moment of doubt or discomfort, is an opportunity to grow stronger, wiser, and more in tune with your body's innate wisdom. Embrace the process with curiosity and self-compassion, knowing that each small victory – whether it's making it through your first 16-hour fast or discovering a new sense of clarity and focus – is a testament to your resilience and adaptability.

Fasting is not just about changing your relationship with food; it's about reclaiming your power and agency in all areas of your life. As you learn to listen to your body's signals, to distinguish between true hunger and emotional cravings, you'll develop a deeper trust in yourself and your ability to navigate life's challenges with grace and intention.

So start small, be patient with yourself, and celebrate every step forward on this path to greater health, happiness, and self-awareness. Know that you are capable of extraordinary things, and that by committing to this journey of self-discovery, you are planting the seeds for a life of boundless energy, vitality, and joy.

May your fasting journey be a catalyst for profound transformation – not just in your body, but in your mind, your heart, and your very way of being in the world. And may you emerge from this experience with a renewed sense of purpose, a deeper connection to your highest self, and a radiant, unstoppable zest for life that inspires everyone around you.

Here's to the adventure of a lifetime – let's begin!

Key Questions To Explore Before You Begin

Please take the time to answer this questions prior to beginning your fasting practice.

1. What do you hope to gain from fasting?

_____

_____

_____

_____

_____

_____

_____

_____

2. What aspects of your current lifestyle do you wish to transform through the alchemy of fasting?

3. What habits or patterns are keeping you feeling stuck or stagnant?

4. How can the practice of fasting support your overall vision for a balanced and fulfilled life?

_____

_____

_____

_____

_____

5. How does this balanced and fulfilled life look like?

_____

_____

_____

_____

_____

6. What challenges and triumphs do you expect from fasting, and how could they contribute to your overall personal development?

Guiding Questions While You Fast

On Hunger

1. Are you experiencing a sudden, urgent craving, or has your hunger gradually intensified over time?

Consider whether your hunger might be a response to emotional stress or a natural physical need. Emotional hunger is sudden and strong; physical hunger is slow and steady.

2. Are you craving a specific type of food or would any food satisfy your hunger?

Reflect on whether your hunger is driven by an emotional craving for a particular item, like chocolate, or a general physical need to eat. Emotional hunger seeks specific foods; physical hunger accepts any food in general.

3. Do you feel hunger as a craving in your mind and mouth, or as a rumble in your stomach?

Think about whether your hunger is a response to seeing food and thinking about it, or a physical need signaled by your body. Emotional hunger is felt in the head, physical hunger is felt in the gut.

4. How do you feel after eating—guilty or at peace?

Reflect on whether these feelings might indicate if you're eating due to emotional triggers or actual physical hunger. Eating to meet physical needs seldom leaves us with the guilt hangover that accompanies meals consumed for emotional reasons.

On Exercise

1. How long has it been since your last meal when you decide to exercise?

Reflect on how this timing affects your energy levels and performance. Think of the type of fuel (glucose or ketones) you used during your workout and how it felt in your body.

2. Was your workout anaerobic or aerobic?

Reflect on how you felt during the exercise, considering whether ketones or glucose fueled your performance. Try the same workout using the other fuel and compare.

3. How much did you enjoy your workout?

Reflect on what elements contributed to your enjoyment or lack thereof.

5. What physical sensations did you experience one to two hours after your workout?

Reflect on how these sensations might inform your understanding of your body's response to exercise in a fasted state.

On Eating

1. How satisfied are you with what you ate?

Reflect on the factors that contributed to your satisfaction or dissatisfaction with your meal.

2. Was your recent decision to eat driven by emotional or physical hunger?

Consider the cues that led you to eat.

3. Are you experiencing symptoms like acid reflux, gas, burping, or an upset stomach?

Reflect on which foods might have caused these issues. Was it a single food or a combination?

4. When did you feel the hungriest today? Was this peak hunger close to your scheduled feeding window?

Reflect on whether adjusting your feeding window might better accommodate your natural hunger cues.

On Sleep

1. How many hours did you sleep last night, and did you feel it was enough?

Reflect on how refreshed you felt upon waking up.

2. How many times did you wake up last night, and what were the reasons?

Consider how often you needed to use the bathroom and reflect on the timing of your last drink and meal before bed. Should you adjust your eating or drinking schedule to minimize disruptions to your sleep?

Bibliography

1. **Brewer, Judson.**
   2016. "*A Simple Way to Break a Bad Habit.*" TED Talks, February. https://www.ted.com/talks/judson_brewer_a_simple_way_to_break_a_bad_habit/transcript?language=en.

2. **Clegg, Jennifer.**
   2024. "*Four Easy, Effective Ways to Distinguish Emotional Hunger.*" LinkedIn. Accessed April 10, 2024. https://www.linkedin.com/pulse/four-easy-effective-ways-distinguish-emotional-hunger-clegg-lpc/.

3. **Galluzzi, Lorenzo, José Manuel Bravo-San Pedro, Beth Levine, David C. Rubinsztein, and Guido Kroemer.**
   2019. "*Autophagy: Cancer, Other Pathologies, Inflammation, Immunity, Infection, and Aging.*" Annual Review of Cancer Biology 3: 11-32. https://www.ncbi.nlm.nih.gov/pmc/articles/PMC6451361/.

4. **Gudden, Jip, Alejandro Arias Vasquez, and Mirjam Bloemendaal.**
   2021. "*The Effects of Intermittent Fasting on Brain and Cognitive Function.*" Nutrients 13, no. 3166. https://doi.org/10.3390/nu13093166. Accessed April 2024.

5. **Hall, Kevin D., and Scott Kahan.**
   2018. "*Maintenance of Lost Weight and Long-Term Management of Obesity.*" Medical Clinics of North America 102, no. 1: 183–97. https://doi.

org/10.1016/j.mcna.2017.08.012.

6. **Harari, Yuval N**.
   2014. *Sapiens: A Brief History of Humankind*. New York: Harper.

7. **Haupt, Sandra, Max L. Eckstein, Alina Wolf, Rebecca T. Zimmer, Nadine B. Wachsmuth, and Othmar Moser.**
   2021. *"Eat, Train, Sleep—Retreat? Hormonal Interactions of Intermittent Fasting, Exercise and Circadian Rhythm."* Biomolecules 11, no. 4 (April): 516. https://doi.org/10.3390/biom11040516.

8. **Hill, Deborah, Mark Conner, Faye Clancy, Rachael Moss, Sarah Wilding, Matt Bristow, and Daryl B. O'Connor.**
   2022. *"Stress and Eating Behaviours in Healthy Adults: A Systematic Review and Meta-Analysis."* Health Psychology Review 16, no. 2: 280-304. https://doi.org/10.1080/17437199.2021.1923406.

9. **Klempel, Monica C., Surabhi Bhutani, Marian Fitzgibbon, Sally Freels, and Krista A. Varady.**
   2010. *"Dietary and Physical Activity Adaptations to Alternate Day Modified Fasting: Implications for Optimal Weight Loss."* Nutrition Journal 9, no. 35. https://doi.org/10.1186/1475-2891-9-35.

10. **Longo, Valter D., and Satchidananda Panda.**
    2016. *"Fasting, Circadian Rhythms, and Time-Restricted Feeding in Healthy Lifespan."* Cell Metabolism 23, no. 6 (June 14): 1048-1059. https://doi.org/10.1016/j.cmet.2016.06.001.

11. **MacCormack, Jennifer K., and Kristen A. Lindquist.**

    2019. *"Feeling Hangry? When Hunger Is Conceptualized as Emotion."* Emotion 19, no. 2: 301-319. https://doi.org/10.1037/emo0000422.

12 **Pilon, Brad.**

    2007. *Eat Stop Eat.* USA: Self-Published.

13. **Stevenson, R. J., J. Bartlett, M. Wright, A. Hughes, B. J. Hill, S. Saluja, and H. M. Francis.**

    2023. *"The Development of Interoceptive Hunger Signals."* Developmental Psychobiology 65: e22374. https://doi.org/10.1002/dev.22374.

14. **Swami, V., S. Hochstoger, E. Kargl, and S. Stieger.**

    2022. *"Hangry in the Field: An Experience Sampling Study on the Impact of Hunger on Anger, Irritability, and Affect."* PLoS ONE 17(7): e0269629. https://doi.org/10.1371/journal.pone.0269629.

15. **The Nutrition Source.**

    "Diet Review: Ketogenic Diet for Weight Loss." Harvard T.H. Chan School of Public Health. Last accessed April 10, 2024. https://www.hsph.harvard.edu/nutritionsource/healthy-weight/diet-reviews/ketogenic-diet/.

16. **Tinsley, Grant M., M. Lane Moore, Austin J. Graybeal, Antonio Paoli, Youngdeok Kim, Joaquin U. Gonzales, John R. Harry, Trisha A. VanDusseldorp, Devin N. Kennedy, and Megan R. Cruz.**

2019. *"Time-Restricted Feeding Plus Resistance Training in Active Females: A Randomized Trial."* The American Journal of Clinical Nutrition 110, no. 3: 628-640. https://doi.org/10.1093/ajcn/nqz126.

17. **Van Proeyen, Karen, Karolina Szlufcik, Henri Nielens, Monique Ramaekers, and Peter Hespel.**

    2011. *"Beneficial Metabolic Adaptations Due to Endurance Exercise Training in the Fasted State."* Journal of Applied Physiology 110, no. 1: 236-245. Accessed April 2024. https://www.ncbi.nlm.nih.gov/pmc/articles/PMC3253005/.

18. **Vasiliev, Vladimir.**

    2006. *Let Every Breath: Secrets of the Russian Breath Masters.* Toronto, Canada: Russian Martial Art.

19. **Wilhelmi de Toledo, Françoise, Franziska Grundler, Cesare R. Sirtori, and Massimiliano Ruscica.**

    2020. *"Unravelling the Health Effects of Fasting: A Long Road from Obesity Treatment to Healthy Life Span Increase and Improved Cognition."* Annals of Medicine 52, no. 5: 147-161. https://doi.org/10.1080/07853890.2020.1770849.

Made in United States
Troutdale, OR
12/08/2024